Migraine

Edited by Wojciech Kozubski

Published in London, United Kingdom

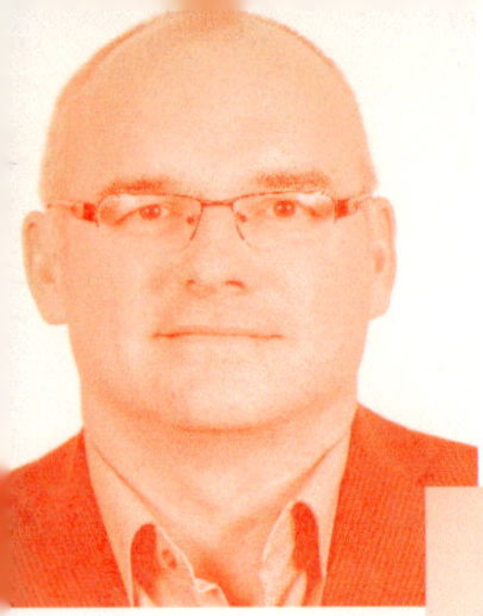
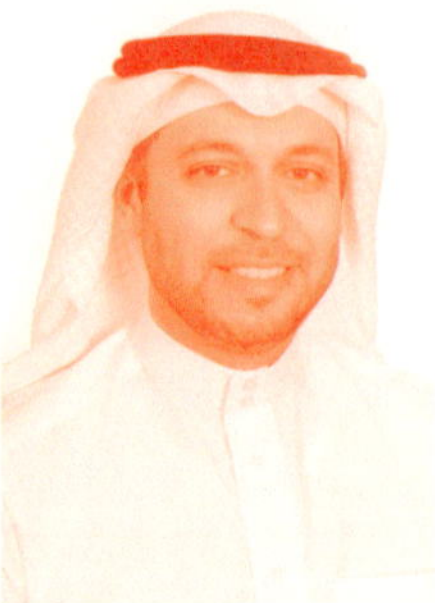
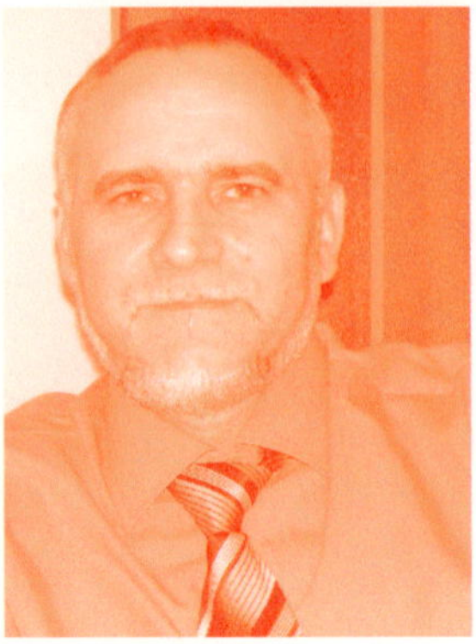
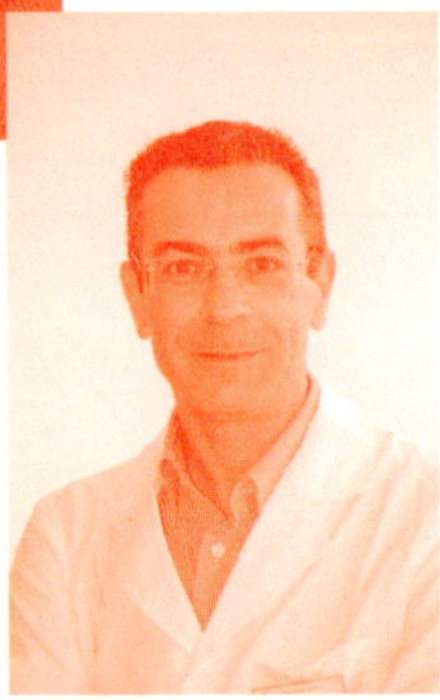
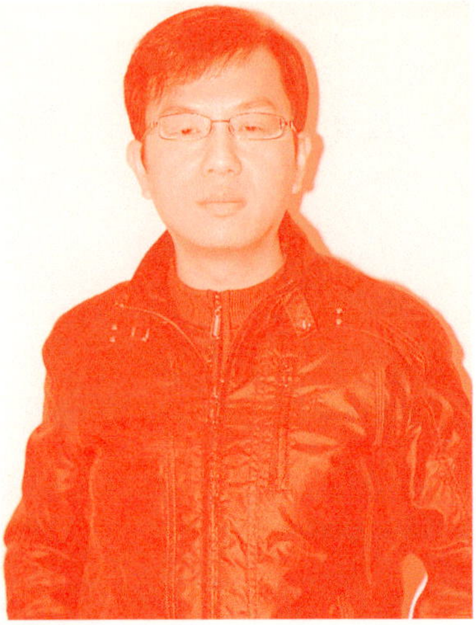
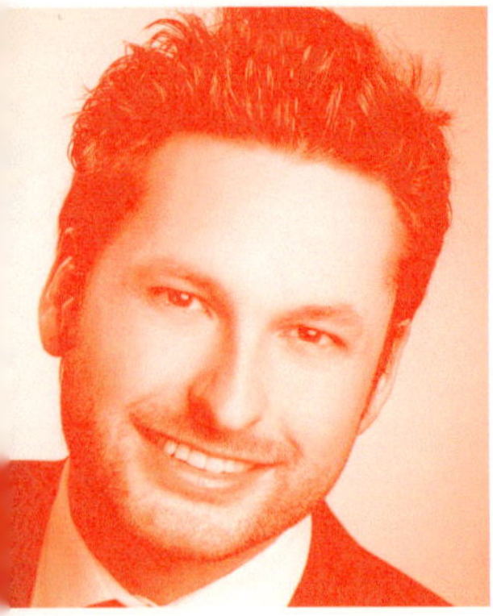
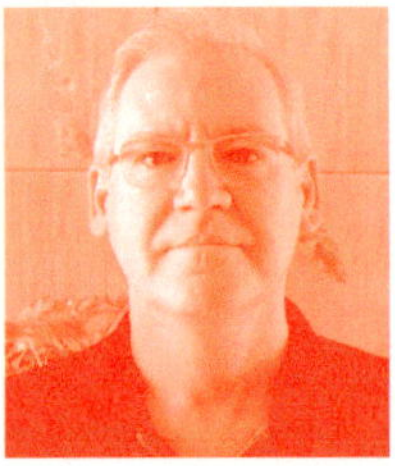

IntechOpen

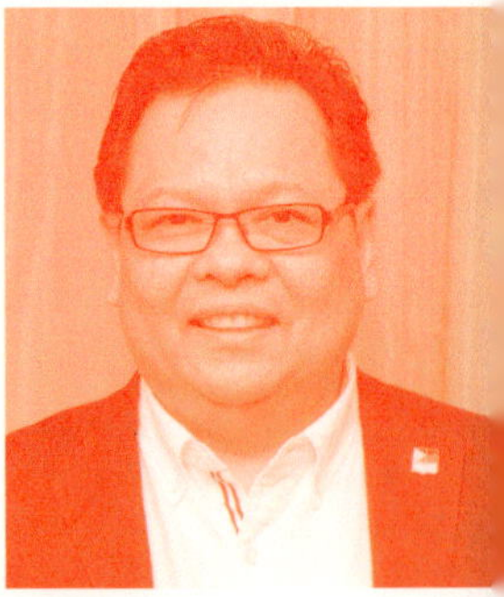
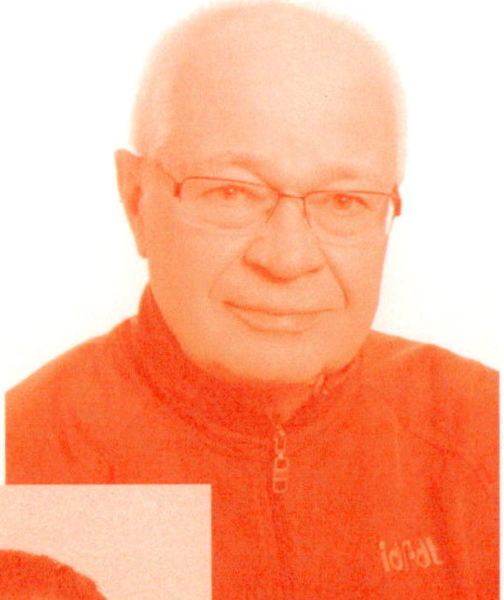
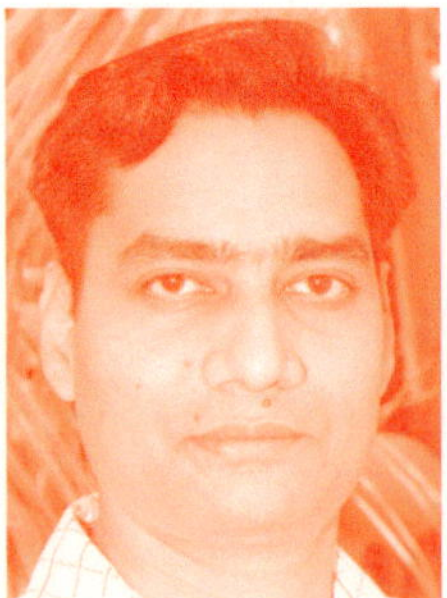
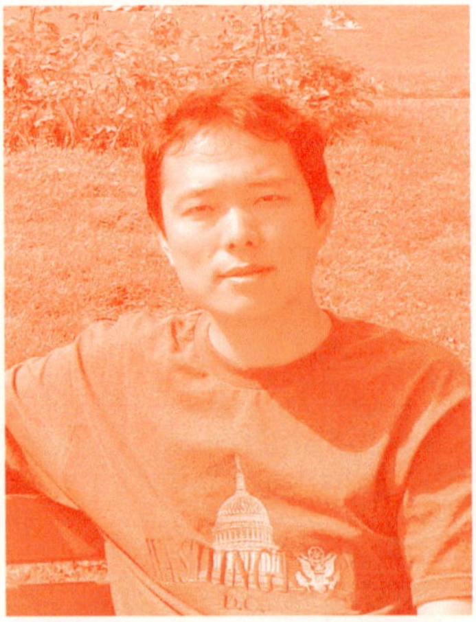
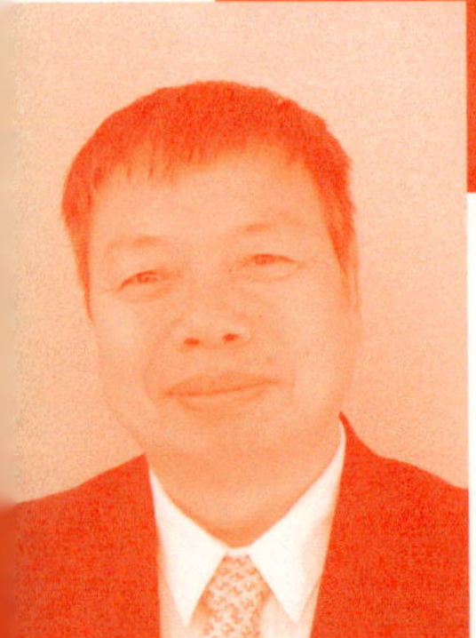
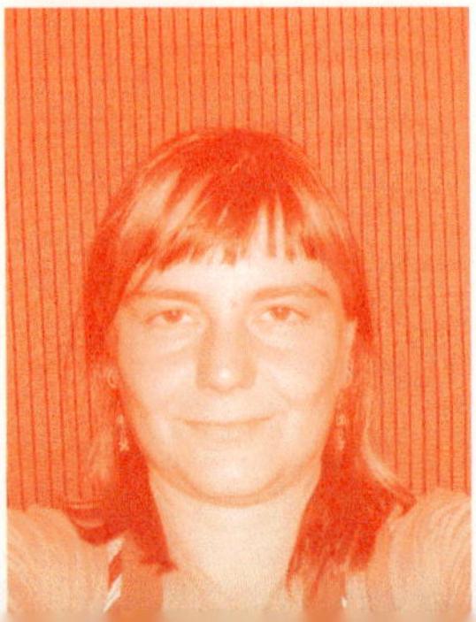

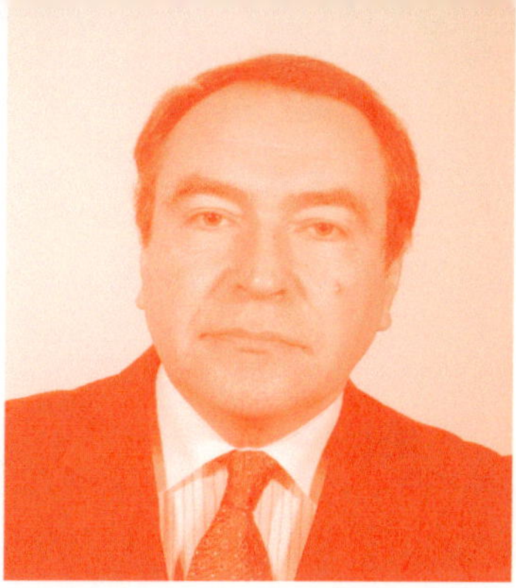

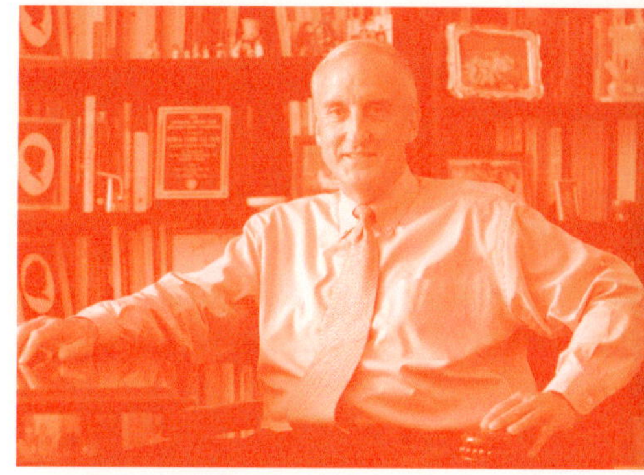

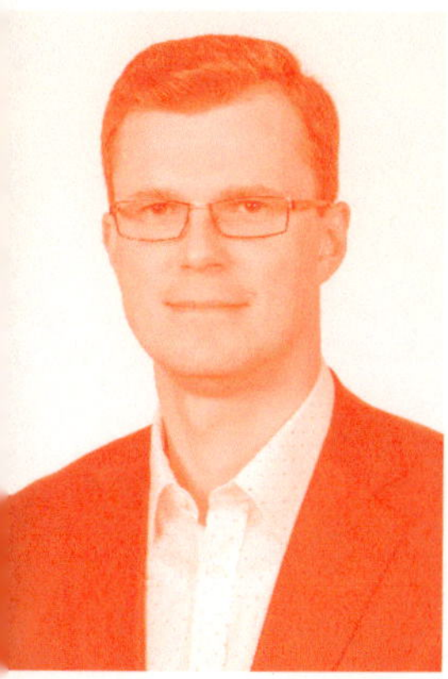

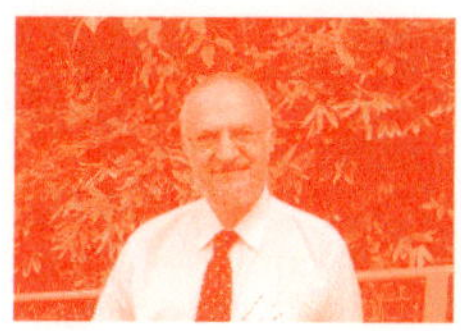

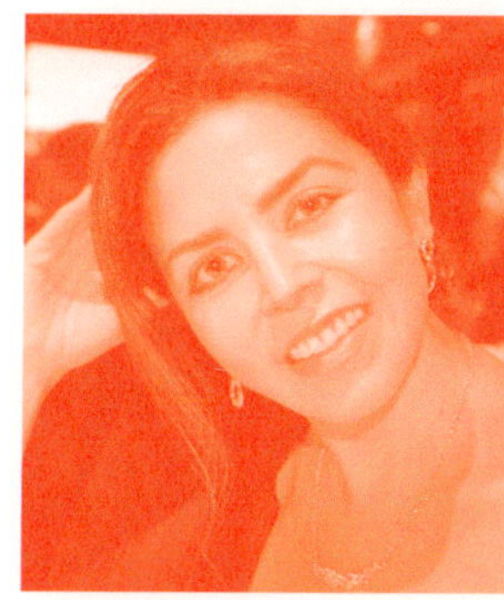

Supporting open minds since 2005

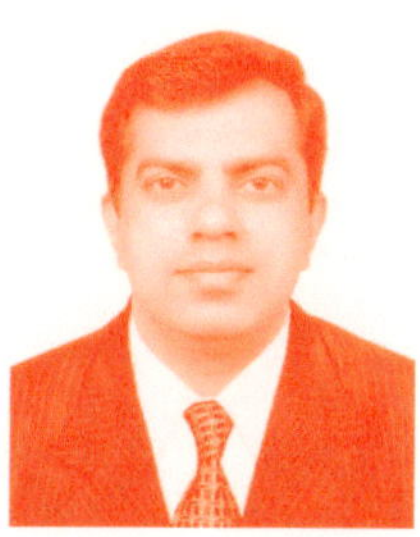

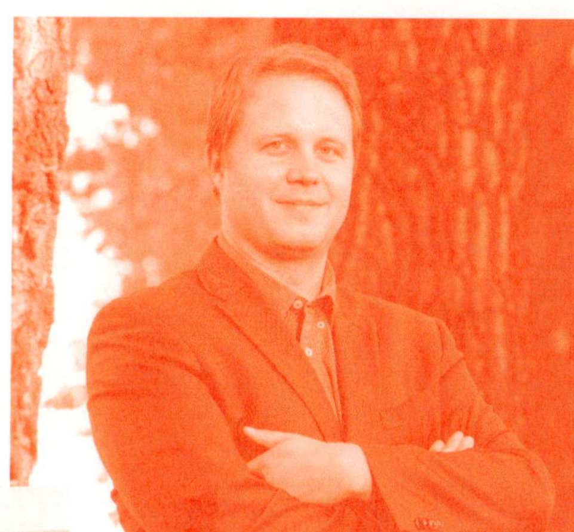

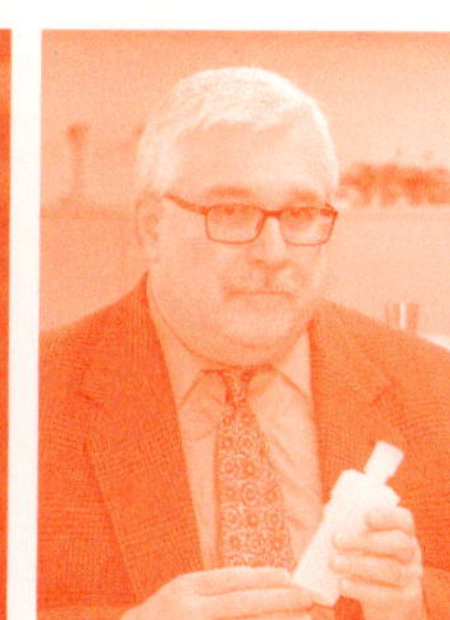

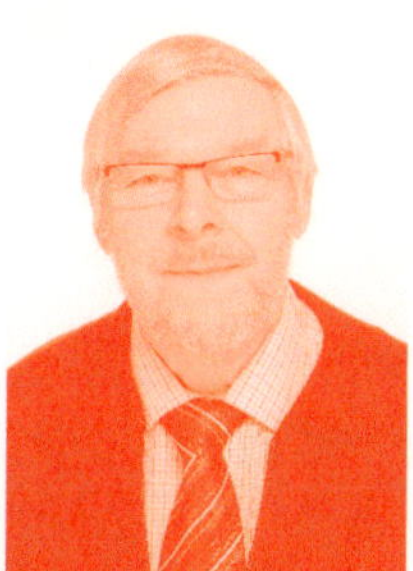

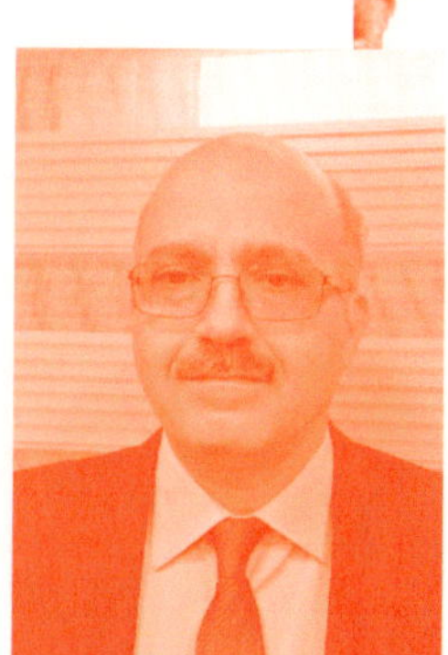

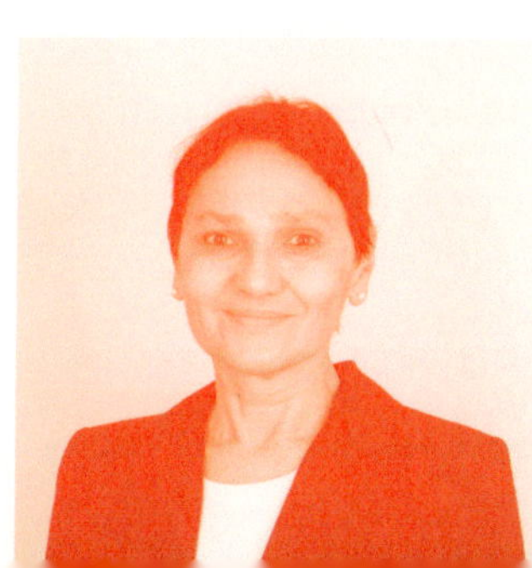

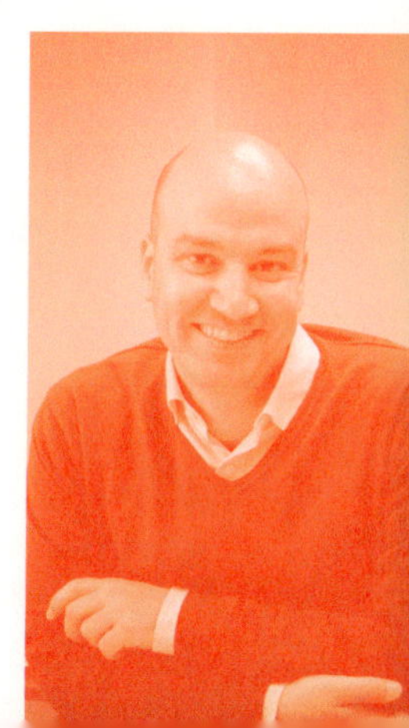

Migraine
http://dx.doi.org/10.5772/intechopen.87586
Edited by Wojciech Kozubski

Contributors
Francesco Simonacci, Edoardo Raposio, Nicolò Bertozzi, Gianluigi Lago, Fante Carlo, Giuseppe Sanese, Balaji Ommurugan, Vanishree Rao, Marcos Antonio Da Silva Cristovam, Daniel Albiero Piélak, Julia Deitos, Júlia Natsumi Hashimoto, Lorena Vaz Meleiro Lopes, Luísa Manfredin Vila, Diana Obelieniene, Ruta Pestininkaite, Daiva Rastenyte, Dimos-Dimitrios Mitsikostas, Theodoros Mavridis, Christina Deligianni, Marianthi Breza, Fayyaz Ahmed, Dhruv Bansal, Pritesh Pranay, Wojciech Kozubski, Izabela Domitrz

First published in London, United Kingdom, 2020 by IntechOpen
IntechOpen is the global imprint of INTECHOPEN LIMITED, registered in England and Wales, registration number: 11086078, 5 Princes Gate Court, London, SW7 2QJ, United Kingdom
Printed in Croatia

British Library Cataloguing-in-Publication Data
A catalogue record for this book is available from the British Library

Additional hard and PDF copies can be obtained from orders@intechopen.com

Migraine
Edited by Wojciech Kozubski
p. cm.
Print ISBN 978-1-83962-409-4
Online ISBN 978-1-83962-410-0
eBook (PDF) ISBN 978-1-83962-411-7

For EU product safety concerns:
IN TECH d.o.o., Prolaz Marije Krucifikse Kozulić 3, 51000 Rijeka, Croatia, info@intechopen.com or visit our website at intechopen.com.

Meet the editor

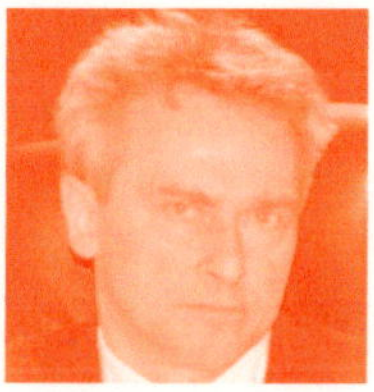

Prof. Wojciech Kozubski, MD, PhD is the Head of the Department of Neurology, University of Medical Sciences in Poznan, Poland. He graduated from Medical School in Lodz in 1980. In 1983 he received his PhD and in 2002, his professorship. From 1987 to 1991, he was awarded a scholarship from the Academic Unit of Neuroscience, University of London, Department of Neurology, University of Tel-Aviv and the Department of Neurology, University of Trondheim. He is an author and co-author of over 300 papers concerning the migraine and related headaches, stroke, and dementia. He is the editor of the handbook of clinical neurology for neurologists, the handbook for medical students, monographs on brain tumours, affective diseases of nervous system and therapy in neurology. From 2011 to 2014, he was the President of the Polish Neurological Society.

Contents

Preface

Dear Readers,

A migraine, as described over 6 thousand years ago, is one of the oldest described entities, not only in neurology but in all medicine. It is also one of the most common diseases worldwide, including 11-13% of the Western population. Despite years of research and efforts, the disease still remains a mystery in its aetiology and pathophysiology with comparatively modest therapeutic results.

Probably, because of that the migraine is still a developing field both in laboratory research and in clinical neurology, involving a number of research workers in many countries. In recent years new hopes and, what is more important, possibilities have come into sight on therapeutic horizons. The monoclonal antibodies developed against the CGRP complex had high prophylactic effectiveness, especially in the chronic type of the disease.

This book covers the most important fields in migraine study and touches on the essential problems of symptomatology, pathophysiology, and therapy of the disease.

The authors of the respective chapters are widely recognized experts in clinical neurology, strictly confined to migraine and headache problems.

The book may serve as invaluable help in the diagnosis and therapy of migraines for all the specialists that might be interested in headache problems, i.e. neurologists, psychiatrists, internal medicine doctors and many others.

The special attention was confined to specific problems in 'migrainology' and related fields, as the chronic type of the disease, contemporary modes of migraine treatment, and that seems to be especially important nowadays, as it is still a troublesome problem of medical overused headache.

Wojciech Kozubski MD, PhD
Professor,
Poznań University of Medical Sciences,
Poland

Section 1

Introduction

Chapter 1

Introductory Chapter: Migraine in Post-Triptan Era – New Therapeutic Horizons

Wojciech Kozubski and Izabela Domitrz

1. Introduction

Migraine is described as a chronic, most probably genetically determined disease, in vast majority of patients characterized by the occurrence of headache attacks. The bouts of headache are accompanied by specific symptoms and signs as nausea—in majority of patients and vomiting—in almost half of them, as well as photophobia and phonophobia [1]. Since they left untreated, the attacks last—in adult patient—from 4 hours up to 3 days. The onset of the disease falls between 18 and 35 years and migraine is regarded as a life-long condition, however it may present a different clinical face in different period of patient's life as far as frequency and severity of the attacks are concerned. In general, migraine is more than twice more common in adult women (approx. 15% of general population) than in adult men—roughly 6% of the population [2], especially in the period of highest occurrence. However, relations and proportions might be entirely different in childhood and senescence—approximately the same percentage of young boys suffer from migraine as girls [3] and the disease is almost three times more common among elderly men than postmenopausal women [4].

The vast majority of the patients usually experience the moderate and/or severe pain intensity during attacks. It results in the fact that almost three-quarters of migraine victims present highly diminished effectiveness during disease attack [5]. It means the effective treatment of each single attack plays a decisive role in the reduction of both biological (i.e. pain, accompanying symptoms), social and economic aspects of the disease.

2. Triptans

For a long time specific and selective 5-$HT_{1B/1D}$ receptor agonists—a class of drugs called triptans (including sumatriptan, zolmitriptan, naratriptan, rizatriptan, almotriptan, eletriptan, and frovatriptan)—have been used as an effective and relatively safe measures against migraine attacks, regarded as almost the drugs of choice in migraine episodes [6, 7]. The drugs were especially recommended in patients with attacks poorly responded to NSAIDs or in whom NSAIDs were contraindicated. What is more—the fewer side effects were associated with triptans than in other anti-migraine drugs, and triptans were more effective at aborting migraine bouts [8]. However, during the years of triptan administration, it was noticed, that these group of drugs, even used in proper dose and manner are ineffective in some 16–18% of migraine victims [9]. What is more the side effects of triptans

IntechOpen

(coronary-like pain symptoms) appeared dangerous and strictly unacceptable for quite a percentage of patients [10]—in fact, triptans are contraindicated in most cardiovascular diseases. In these situation the strong need of new—effective and especially cardiac—safe migraine killers—became obvious.

3. After triptans

The next selective drugs tried in abortive treatment in migraine were ditans—a class of molecules that selectively bind to 5-HT_{1F} receptors. The ditans are not encountered in vessels, being widespread in CNS, especially in brain stem, hampering the increased trigeminal system activity during migraine attack [11]. After the years of clinical studies, one of these molecules—lasmiditan, after first—relatively positive trials [12]—finally—has been approved by the FDA for the acute treatment of migraine with or without aura in adults [13].

Also the next seemingly promising group—gepants, calcitonin-gene related peptide (CGRP) receptor antagonist—after first enthusiastic results concerning the efficacy of the first generation of antagonist—telcagepant [14] or ubrogepant [15], were the subject of more detailed debates and considerations. The main reason for the doubts was their accented hepatotoxicity [16]. Eventually, the FDA has approved an orally disintegrating tablet formulation of rimegepant [17], that was the second, after ubrogepant, oral drug of this group, available in anti-migraine armamentarium. We still waiting for the final results and the potential approval of the next two molecules from second gepants generation, i.e. atogepant, vazegepant.

4. Monoclonal antibodies against CGRP and the CGRP receptor as new-generation drugs for migraine treatment

Monoclonal antibodies (mAbs) developed against CGRP receptor (as erenumab) or CGRP molecule itself (namely—fremanezumab, galcanezumab, and eptinezumab) were the next big hope in therapeutic attitude to migraine. The drugs of these group exert strong inhibiting effect on CGRP release during migraine attack, thus hampering its vasodilative effect [18, 19]. The results of many registered pharmacoclinical studies/trials showed both effectiveness and safety of these drugs, that reduced both the number of migraine episodes, days with headache and administration of acute headache killers per month in migraineurs. The next advantages of these group were very convenient, patient-friendly dose regimen (once a four weeks) and—as it looks now—the absence of serious side effect [20, 21]. It seems that relatively fast onset of action (in the first month of implementation), high efficacy, and good tolerability make this class of drugs the real revolution in migraine treatment [22, 23] compared with that of ergotamine introduction (in 1927) or the first triptans in 1990. In fact, they are the second characteristic molecule—after methysergide—targeting the most specific mechanism of migraine attacks. This group of drugs showed effectiveness both in episodic and chronic migraine—and what is more, also, in migraine-like episodes in patients with cerebral autosomal dominant arteriopathy with subcortical infarcts and leukoencephalopathy (CADASIL), that is quite a phenomenon [24].

We do hope that in time and gaining more experience with these group of antimigraine drugs, monoclonal antibodies against CGRP complex will become the first-line treatment of the disease.

Author details

Wojciech Kozubski[1*] and Izabela Domitrz[2]

1 Department of Neurology, Charles Marcinkowski University of Medical Sciences in Poznan, Poland

2 Department of Neurology, Faculty of Medical Sciences, Medical University of Warsaw, Poland

*Address all correspondence to: wkozubski@ump.edu.pl

References

[1] Ludwig J, Bartsch T, Wasner G, Baron R. Autonomic dysfunction in migraines. In: Olesen J, Goadsby P, Ramadan NM, Tfelt- Hansen P, Welch KMA, editors. The Headaches. 3rd ed. Philadelphia: Lippnicott Williams & Wilkins; 2006. pp. 377-384

[2] Lipton RB, Bigal ME, Diamond M, Freitag F, Reed ML, Stewart WF. Migraine prevalence, disease burden, and the need for preventive therapy. Neurology. 2007;**68**:343-349

[3] Rasmussen BK. Epidemiology of migraine. In: Olesen J, Goadsby P, Ramadan NM, Tfelt- Hansen P, Welch KMA, editors. The Headaches. 3rd ed. Philadelphia: Lippnicott Williams & Wilkins; 2006. pp. 235-242

[4] Prencipe M, Gasini AR, Ferretti C. Prevalence of headache in an elderly population: Attack frequency, disability. and use of medication. J Neurol Neurosurg Psychiatry. 2001;**70**:377-381

[5] Edmeads J, Mackell JA. The economic impact of migraine: An analysis of direct and indirect costs. Headache. 2002;**42**:501-509

[6] Goadsby PJ. Serotonin 51B/1D receptor agonists in migraine. CNS Drugs. 1998;**10**:271-286

[7] Lipton RB, Bigal ME, Rush SR, Yenkosky JP, Liberman JN, Bartleson JD, et al. Practice patterns among neurologists. Neurology. 2004;**62**:1926-1931

[8] Cameron C, Shannon K, Shu-Ching H, Murphy M, et al. Triptans in the Acute Treatment of Migraine: A Systematic Review and Network Meta-Analysis. Headache. 2015;**55**(Suppl. 4): 221-235

[9] Ferrari MD. Migraine. The Lancet. 1998;**351**:1043-1051

[10] Thorlund K, Mills EJ, Wu P, Ramos E, Chatterjee A, Druyts E, et al. Comparative efficacy of triptans for the abortive treatment of migraine: A multiple treatment comparison meta-analysis. Cephalalgia. 2014;**34**:258-267

[11] Jamieson DG. The safety of triptans in the treatment of patients with migraine. The American Journal of Medicine. 2002;**112**:135-140

[12] Vila-Pueyo M, Strother L, Page K, et al. Lasmiditan inhibits trigeminovascular nociceptive transmission. Cephalalgia. 2016;**36**:152

[13] https://www.fda.gov/news-events/press-announcements/fda-approves-new-treatment-patients-migraine.

[14] Farkkila M, Diener HC, Geraud G, et al. Efficacy and tolerability of lasmiditan, an oral 5-HT(1F) receptor agonist, for the acute treatment of migraine: A phase 2 randomized, placebo-controlled, parallel-group, dose-ranging study. Lancet Neurology. 2012;**11**:405-413

[15] Ho TW, Ferrari MD, Dodick DW, et al. Efficacy and tolerability of MK-0974 (telcagepant), a new oral antagonist of calcitonin gene-related peptide receptor, compared with zolmitriptan for acute migraine: A randomized, placebo-controlled, parallel-treatment trial. Lancet. 2008;**372**:2115-2123

[16] Voss T, Lipton RB, Dodick DW, et al. A phase IIb randomized, double-blind, placebo-controlled trial of ubrogepant for the acute treatment of migraine. Cephalalgia. 2016;**36**:887-898

[17] Rimegepant (Nurtec ODT) for Acute Treatment of Migraine. Journal of the American Medical Association. 2020;**324**(9):890-891. DOI: 10.1001/jama.2020.8493

[18] Moreno-Ajona D, Perez-Rodriguez A, Goadsby PJ. Gepants, calcitonin-gene related peptide (CGRP) receptor antagonist: What could be their role in migraine treatment. Current Opinion in Neurology. 2020;**33**:309-315

[19] Russo AF. Calcitonin gene-related peptide (CGRP): A new target for migraine. Annual Review of Pharmacology and Toxicology. 2015;**55**:533-552

[20] Moskowitz MA. Pathopysiology of headache – Past and present. Headache. 2007;**47**(suppl. 1):S58-S63

[21] Sun H, Dodick DW, Silberstein S, et al. Safety and efficacy of AMG 334 for prevention of episodic migraine: A randomized, double-blind, placebo-controlled, phase 2 trial. Lancet Neurol. 2016;**15**:382-390

[22] Silberstein SD, Dodick DW, Bigal ME, et al. Fremanezumab for the preventive treatment of chronic migraine. The New England Journal of Medicine. 2017;**377**:2113-2122

[23] Skljarevski V, Oakes TM, Zhang Q, et al. Effect of different doses of galcanezumab vs placebo for episodic migraine prevention: A randomized clinical trial. JAMA Neurology. 2018;**75**:187-193

[24] Goldstein ED, Badi MK, Meschia JM. Treating chronic migraine in CADASIL with calcitonin gene-related peptide receptor antagonism. Neurology Clinical Practice. 2019. DOI: https://doi.org/10.1212/CPJ.0000000000000651

Section 2

Advances in Migraine Therapy

Chapter 2

Recent Advances in Migraine Therapy

Balaji Ommurugan and Vanishree Rao

Abstract

Migraine characterized by recurrent headache episodes presents with aura or without. Various treatment modalities ranging from 5-HT1B/1D agonists, non-steroidal anti-inflammatory drugs (NSAIDs), to steroids are available for acute treatment of migraine. Prophylaxis for chronic cases usually encompasses β blockers, calcium channel blockers, and antiepileptics. Many nutraceutical preparations are helpful in migraine, including riboflavin and vitamin B_{12}. This review focuses on the newer agents available for treatment of migraine with some insights into their clinical trials.

Keywords: headache, nutraceutical, prophylaxis, triptans, cortical spreading depression

1. Introduction

The word "migraine" comes from the Greek ἡμικρανία (*hemikrania*), "pain on one side of the head"; ἡμι- (*hemi-*), "half"; and κρανίον (*kranion*), "skull." The disorder may also be described as a vascular headache associated with changes in the size of the arteries within and outside the brain [1]. It is usually accompanied by a plethora of comorbidities influencing its clinical expression and complicating its treatment, making migraine a chronic and debilitating neurological disorder. It is a polygenetic disease with high susceptibility to epigenetic factors affecting millions of people worldwide. This is mainly because of changes in hormonal levels. It is estimated that up to 15% of people suffer from migraine worldwide with 1.4–2.2% affected by the chronic form of the disease [2, 3]. Global data shows the prevalence of migraine increasing during adolescence with peaks in midlife and the prevalence declining rapidly after 50 years. Migraine presents as headache and visual, auditory, olfactory, and cutaneous stimuli hypersensitivity along with nausea and vomiting [4]. Both environmental and genetic factors play a role in the development of migraine with more than two third of cases having familial history [5]. Boys are more affected than girls before puberty, but women are more affected than men as age increases [6].

2. Signs and symptoms

Migraine is self-limiting, usually presenting as recurrent severe headache. It is associated with autonomic symptoms. It presents with aura in 15–30% and without aura in the rest [7]. Migraine varies from person to person with respect to severity of pain, duration of attack, and its frequency. A migraine lasting longer than 72 h is termed status migrainosus. Different phases of migraine include the prodrome, the aura, the pain, and the postdrome. The prodromal phase occurs hours before the headache in 60% of patients, the aura usually precedes headache in 15–20%, severe headache occurs in the pain phase, and the postdromal phase usually follows the attack of migraine [8].

3. The pathophysiology of migraine

The best solutions to medical conditions come only from understanding the pathophysiology of the disease state. As per Wolff's vascular theory, vascular constriction leading to hypoperfusion of the cortex later followed by vascular dilation was put forward as the main pathophysiological mechanism. Currently neurovascular hypothesis involving the trigeminovascular system is considered. Another hypothesis includes mutations of neuronal calcium channels, leading to hypersensitivity, resulting in migraine attacks. It is also postulated that increased dopaminergic activity in the thalamus/hypothalamus causing modulation in central pain pathways also plays a role in migraine attacks. Other mechanisms put forward include cortical spreading depression; release of vasoactive peptides like substance P, calcitonin gene-related peptide (CGRP) from trigeminal neural endings, nitric oxide, and serotonin; excess activation of N-methyl-D-aspartate receptor (NMDA) receptors without modulation by brain stem pain centers due to dysfunction of these centers; overactivity of excitatory neurotransmitters like aspartate and glutamate causing neuronal excitability; and finally neurogenic inflammation which play an important role in migraine attack development [9–12].

4. Treatment of migraine

It can be divided into treatment of acute attacks and treatment of chronic migraine. As per the US consortium (2000), recommended guidelines [13] for treatment of acute migraine include pharmacological and non-pharmacological modalities as shown in **Table 1**.

1. Specific treatment
a. Triptans
b. Ergot and its derivatives
2. Nonspecific treatment
a. Antiemetics
b. NSAIDs and nonnarcotic analgesics
c. Narcotics/opiate analgesics

Table 1.
Treatment of acute migraine attacks.

5. Specific treatment

5.1 Triptans

Triptans are selective agonists of 5-HT1B and 5-HT1D receptors. The mechanism of action includes intracranial vessel vasoconstriction (5-HT1B), peripheral neuronal inhibition (5-HT1D), and presynaptic dorsal horn stimulation (5-HT1D), producing second-order brain stem neuronal inhibition. Triptans influence the function

Drugs	Half life	Maximum daily dose
Group 1: fast-acting triptans		
Sumatriptan	3 h	200 mg oral 40 mg intranasal 12 mg subcutaneous
Rizatriptan	2–3 h	30 mg (15 mg if on propranolol)
Almotriptan	3–4 h	25 mg
Zolmitriptan	3 h	Two tablets or 10 mg maximum oral daily dose. Two sprays or 10 mg intranasal
Eletriptan	4 h	80 mg
Group 2: slow-acting triptans		
Frovatriptan	26 h	7.5 mg
Naratriptan	6 h	5 mg

Table 2.
Triptan characteristics.

of 5-hydroxytryptamine 1F (5-HT1F) receptors and enhance descending inhibitory pain pathways. Triptans reduce—to a considerable extent—pain severity in 2 h as per randomized controlled trials. Oral formulations are usually preferred over other formulations, but 6 mg subcutaneous injection of sumatriptan appears to be the most efficacious. As per current evidence, all oral formulations have equal efficacy except for frovatriptan which is less efficacious but has longer duration action. Parenteral preparations are more useful than oral ones, but the choice of medications depends on the clinician as well as the patient. Triptans are the first-line drugs used in acute treatment of moderate-to-severe migraine with the best pain relief occurring if it is taken within 30 min of attack, and a second dose is usually recommended after 2–4 h of initial dose. It is best used in combination with antiemetics and NSAIDs. Adverse effects include serotonin syndrome when used in combination with selective serotonin reuptake inhibitors (SSRIs), and it should be used with caution in patients having ischemic heart disease [14–22]. Characteristics of triptans are summarized in **Table 2**.

6. Ergot and derivatives

Ergots act on multiple receptors including the 5-HT ones, and these account for a robust side effect profile. It is used in acute management of migraine. Side effect includes nausea as well as severe vasoconstriction. It is contraindicated in patients with vascular disease, hepatic problems, renal dysfunction, and hypertension. It is avoided in pregnancy. Dihydroergotamine (DHE) is the only preparation available and is used both parentally and intranasally. Repeated administration of DHE is very effective in refractory cases as well as status migrainosus. It is relatively safe and effective but it requires hospital administration [23–25].

7. Nonspecific treatment

7.1 Nonsteroidal anti-inflammatory drugs

Good quality evidence supports the use of NSAIDs alone or in combination with specific agents. These drugs in combination with antiemetics are comparable to

Drugs	Formulation	Dose used (the dose wording should be mg')
Aspirin	Tablet/oral solution	650–1000 mg
Ketorolac	Tablet	10 mg
Ketoprofen	Capsule	50–75 mg
Ketoprofen-extended release	Capsule	200 mg
Diclofenac potassium	Tablet/powder	50 mg
Meclofenamate	Capsule	50 mg, 100 mg
Ibuprofen	Capsule, tablet, oral suspension	400–1, 0 g
Etodolac	Tablet/capsule	200–500 mg
Naproxen	Tablet	120–550 mg
Naproxen-controlled release	Tablet	750–850 mg maximum

Table 3.
NSAID characteristics.

lower doses of oral triptans. Recently, powdered preparation of diclofenac sodium is approved for treatment of acute attack. Ketorolac, administrated IV, can be used for emergency management of migraine. NSAIDs need to be used with caution in patients with renal toxicity [26–29]. Characteristics of different drugs in this group are summarized in **Table 3**.

7.2 Neuroleptics/antiemetics

Dopamine D2 receptor antagonists can be used alone or in combination to treat headache as well as nausea. It is mostly used in emergency settings and is available in oral, parenteral, and suppository forms, but concerns over extrapyramidal side effects, tardive dyskinesia, and lack of familiarity in their effect on migraine attacks restrict their use to a great extent [30–33]. Characteristics of antiemetics are summarized in **Table 4**.

7.3 Corticosteroids

Steroids are suggested for acute treatment as well as for status migrainosus [34]. They act by reducing the neurogenic inflammation and vasogenic edema and also play an important role in central serotonergic pathways [35]. One study showed that addition of dexamethasone 4 mg per oral to triptans plus NSAID reduces recurrence and is well tolerated in patients with frequent attacks [36, 37].

Drug	Formulation	Dose of migraine
Prochlorperazine	Tablet, suppository	5–10 mg 25 mg
Metoclopramide	Tablet	10 mg
Chlorpromazine	Tablet	10–25 mg
Promethazine	Tablet	25–50 mg
Ondansetron	Tablet, oral disintegrating tablet	4 mg 8 mg

Table 4.
Antiemetic characteristics.

7.4 Opioids

Opioids are the most prescribed drug for acute and rescue therapy in migraine in America. Recent studies have discouraged the use of opioids mainly because it decreases gray matter, increases CGRP release, releases pro-inflammatory peptides, and also causes glutamate receptor activation. It also results in degranulation of mast cells and causes vasodilation. There are many side effects, such as overuse headache and disease progression [38, 39].

8. Newer agents

8.1 CGRP antagonists

Based on migraine pathology theories, trigeminal ganglion activation causes the activation of nociceptive neurons which leads to subsequent release of CGRP. Increased CGRP levels cause plasma protein extrusion, vasodilation, and mast cell degranulation, ultimately leading to neurogenic inflammation. Drugs which antagonize CGRP include olcegepant, telcagepant, and latest approved monoclonal antibodies, namely, erenumab, fremanezumab, and galcanezumab [40]. They prevent binding of endogenous CGRP on its receptors and suppress the stimulation of CGRP on trigeminal ganglion neurons. They inhibit cortical spreading depression [40]. They lack vasoconstrictive effect. Olcegepant is as effective as oral triptans with less cardiovascular side effects such as blood pressure increase and tachycardia. But one major limitation is intravenous dosing. Telcagepant was initially claimed to be as potent as rizatriptan, causing pain relief in 2 h and also sustained pain relief at 24 h and relief of migraine-associated symptoms with overall good tolerability profile, but later the phase II trial was terminated, claiming the drug showed increase in liver transaminases [40]. Eptinezumab is a new drug in this class under trial and is not yet approved by the Food and Drug Administration (FDA).

8.2 Lasmiditan

It is a 5-HT1F receptor agonist. In experimental model, it blocks neurogenic inflammation, decreases c-fos expression, and lacks vasoconstriction. The main postulated mechanisms include inhibition of protein leakage, blockage of secondary trigeminal neuronal activation, and inhibition of neuropeptide release like glutamate. In a double-blind placebo-controlled parallel group study in 512 patients, the oral form and dose of 50, 100, 200, and 400 mg in moderate-to-severe migraine attacks proved that it is as effective as sumatriptan without causing vasoconstriction, but the significant drawback is its major side effects in the central nervous system. Studies also show a great improvement in headache response in 2 h but also show high 24-h headache recurrence rate [41].

8.3 Tezampanel

Tezampanel acts as a competitive antagonist of the α-amino-3-hydroxy-5-methyl-4-isoxazolepropionic acid (AMPA) and kainate receptor (subtype $GluR_5$) of the ionotropic glutamate receptor family. A randomized triple-blind parallel group double-dummy, multicenter trial showed 1.2 mg tezampanel had 69% headache response rate when compared to 6 mg s.c. sumatriptan which had a response rate of 86%. It is effective and well tolerated in migraine. It can be used only via intravenous route. Dasolampanel is an orally bioavailable analog of tezampanel. Both drugs were never marketed [42]. Other newer agents are summarized in **Table 5**.

Newer targets and drugs	Current status
1. Adenosine receptor agonists [43]	• GR79236 and GR190178 • GR79236: carotid vasoconstriction than prejunctional inhibition of CGRP release
2. NXN-188 [44]	• A selective nNOS inhibitor + 5-HT1B/5-HT1D receptor agonist inhibits CGRP release in preclinical animal models
3. LY2951742 [45]	• Monoclonal antibody to CGRP under trial
4. Orexin receptor antagonism [46] (filorexant)	Orexin: trigeminal nociceptive and CSD RCT: failed efficacy
5. TRPV1 antagonism (SB-705498) [47]	• Trigeminal nociceptors: heat- and capsaicin-gated channel TRPV1 • Peripheral and central sensitization of trigeminovascular system
6. Melatonin [48]	• Abnormal levels: decreased inhibitory neurotransmission • Decrease inhibition of release of CGRP
7. P2Y purinergic receptors [49]	• Involved in pain signaling and future receptor target

Table 5.
Newer targets and drugs.

8.4 Prophylaxis

It is indicated when a patient meets the following criteria [50]:

- Four or more migraine days per month.
- Recurring migraines significantly interfere with daily activity.
- Contraindication/failure/overuse—acute therapies.
- Overwhelming costs of acute therapies.
- Uncommon migraine conditions—hemiplegic and basilar migraine.

8.5 Beta blockers

Various beta blockers used are summarized in **Table 6**. The mechanisms by which they act include inhibition of central beta receptors and antagonism of 5-HT1A and 5-HT1B receptors, thereby reducing neuronal excitability. It inhibits nitric oxide (NO) production by blocking inducible nitric oxide synthase and

Drugs	Daily doses
Propranolol	40–400 mg
Nadolol	20–160 mg
Metoprolol	100–200 mg
Atenolol	50–200 mg
Timolol	20–60 mg

Table 6.
Beta blockers and dosage.

Drugs	Comment
1. Flunarizine	• 5–10 mg (bedtime) • Used in Europe
2. Verapamil	• 120–640 mg (bid/tid) • 2 trials have shown efficacy better than placebo but more randomized trials to prove its efficacy [55]

Table 7.
Calcium channel blockers and dosage.

inhibits excitatory activity of glutamate, thereby reducing neuronal activity. They also inhibit kainate-induced currents (synergistic with NMDA blockers) and reduce neuronal activity and also have additional membrane-stabilizing action [51, 52].

8.6 Carvedilol: novel β blocker in migraine

In an open-label trial of 76 patients, a dose of 3.125–6.25 mg twice a week was used, and it was found that 60% of patients had 50% reduction in monthly migraine attack frequency and severity, but in 26% of patients, there was lack of efficacy with the drug [53].

8.7 Calcium channel blockers

It inhibits calcium entry and prevents intoxication of cells exposed to cerebral hypoxia due to cortical spreading depression [54]. Various drugs used are summarized in **Table 7**. Other possible mechanisms include inhibition of 5-HT release, inhibition of neurovascular inflammation, and cortical spreading depression.

9. Antiepileptics

9.1 Divalproex sodium

It is a combination of valproic acid and sodium valproate. It is used at a dose of 500–1500 mg/day. Mechanisms include prolongation of sodium channel inactivation, suppression of calcium-mediated T current, and inhibition of gamma-aminobutyric acid (GABA) transaminase. Adverse effect includes nausea, vomiting, gastrointestinal distress, alopecia, and craniofacial abnormalities in fetus [56].

9.2 Topiramate

Topiramate is a recently approved drug for migraine prophylaxis. Starting dose of 15–25 mg at bedtime and increase 15–25 mg/week [57]. Mechanisms include blocking of the voltage-gated sodium channel and inhibition of activation of AMPA-kainate receptor of glutamate, and it also enhances postsynaptic $GABA_A$ receptor current. Adverse effects include somnolence, fatigue, weight loss, nervousness, and precipitation of renal calculi.

9.3 Tiagabine

It inhibits GABA transporter (GAT-1) and thereby reduces GABA uptake into the neurons and glia. It is still not approved by the FDA. In an open-label trial of

41 patients who failed with treatment of valproates with 4 mg QID, 33/41 patients showed 50% reduction in migraine attacks, and 5 patients showed complete remission in migraine [58].

9.4 Levetiracetam (LCT)

It modifies synaptic release of glutamate/GABA by binding to specific synaptic protein (SV_2A). Anecdotal evidence says prevention of migraine. A 10-week open-label study, evaluating efficacy and safety of LCT for pediatric migraine in a population of 30 children or adolescents aged 6–19 years, showed a reduction in headache frequency and severity [59].

9.5 Zonisamide

It blocks voltage-dependent sodium and T-type calcium channels and decreases glutamate-mediated excitatory neurotransmission. Also, it inhibits excessive NO production and helps in scavenging NO and hydroxyl radicals. In an open-label trial, 33 patients with migraine headache, refractory to other preventive therapies, were given a dose of 100–600 mg every third day. Results showed that 65% of patients had a reduction in frequency of migraine attacks [60].

9.6 Antidepressants

Possible mechanisms include reuptake inhibition of serotonin and noradrenaline, α-adrenergic and NMDA-receptor antagonism, sodium and calcium channel blocking action, and potassium channel activation. Increase in $GABA_B$ receptor action and opioid receptor binding/opioid-mediated effect is another minor action. It reduces inflammation by decreasing prostaglandin (PGE_2) and tumor necrosis factor (TNF-α). Various drugs are summarized in **Table 8**. Venlafaxine is used at a dose of 75–225 mg: a double-blind placebo controlled trial showed that the drug was better than placebo, starting with 37.5 mg extended release tablet/week followed by 75 mg for another week and then 150 mg extended release in the morning [61].

9.7 Drugs acting on renin-angiotensin system

The renin-angiotensin system plays a role in neurogenic inflammation and causes increased susceptibility to oxidative stress. It also causes endothelial dysfunction and neuromodulator in nociception. Lisinopril alters sympathetic activity and inhibits free radical activation. It also increases prostacyclin synthesis and blocks the degradation of bradykinin, substance P, and encephalin. In a double-blind placebo-controlled crossover study, patients aged 19–59 years with migraine were treated with 20 mg Lisinopril for 11 weeks—21% of patients showed 50% reduction in migraine attacks [62]. In a comparative study of candesartan vs

Drugs	Daily doses
Amitriptyline	10–400 mg
Doxepin	10–300 mg
Nortriptyline	10–150 mg
Protriptyline	5–60 mg

Table 8.
Antidepressant dosage.

propranolol for migraine prophylaxis in 72 patients, 43% of patients showed greater than 50% reduction in migraine, and it was equally efficacious to propranolol [63].

9.8 Onabotulinum toxin

It is the FDA-approved drug for prophylaxis of chronic migraine at doses ranged from 155 to 195 IU, and it is injected in seven craniofacial and neck muscles, usually the temporalis. It inhibits neurogenic inflammation by inhibiting the release of nociceptive mediators like glutamate, substance P, and CGRP from the peripheral terminals of the efferent nerves. The analgesic action of onabotulinum toxin is central but yet to be proved. It will effect 3 h after injection and last for at least 7 days. Novel delivery routes such as topical/subcutaneous applications are under research [64].

9.9 H_3 agonists

It is used to limit the excessive inflammatory response through H_3 receptor activation. Drugs include Nα-methylhistamine and investigational drug SCH 50971. Phase III double-blind placebo-controlled trial for 12 weeks in 60 patients with a dose of 1–3 mg twice a week caused a reduction in headache frequency, intensity, and duration in 80% of patients. It helps in reducing the dose of analgesics used [65].

9.10 Tonabersat

Preclinical studies showed inhibition of cortical spreading depression by the drug. It inhibits neurogenic inflammation and also the gap junctional intercellular communication (GJIC) between the neurons and satellite glial cells. Various randomized double-blind parallel group placebo-controlled multicenter studies for acute migraine were tried. There are conflicting reports of headache relief at 2/4 h and reasons are not found. In one study with 40 mg on 39 patients, it was found to be effective for migraine with aura when compared to that without it, reinforcing its inhibitory effect on CSD [66].

10. Nutraceuticals in migraine

10.1 Magnesium

Multiple studies show migraine is associated with low levels of magnesium. It causes an influx of calcium into the neurons, causing glutamate release into the neurons, which results in neuronal activation. The onset and propagation of cortical spreading depression is delayed and decreases. It also causes change in neurotransmitter secretion and intensifies the secretion of substance P. It is used in patients with aura and premenstrual migraine and is used at a dose of 1, 0 g IV and 300–600 mg orally in chelated magnesium (taurate, glycinate, oxide) [67]. Magnesium plus L-carnitine is a newer preparation available.

10.2 Coenzyme Q10 (CoQ)

It promotes electron transfer from complex I and II to cytochrome C and helps in ATP production. It protects the mitochondria from free radical damage. A study of 1478 migraine patients of age range 3–22 years showed low levels of CoQ in 33%

of patients. A randomized controlled trial of 42 patients receiving 100 mg TID for 3 months found it superior to placebo, and 48% of subjects have greater than 50% reduction in migraine attacks [68].

10.3 Riboflavin

It is a cofactor in the Krebs cycle. Abnormal phosphorylation of ADP to ATP is prevented with riboflavin. A randomized controlled trial with 400 mg riboflavin taken daily for 3 months was superior to placebo for reduction of migraine frequency [69]. A randomized controlled trial with 400 mg of riboflavin plus feverfew and low-dose magnesium was comparable to a 25 mg active riboflavin. Greater than 40% of patients showed 50% reduction in migraine attacks [70].

10.4 Vitamin B_{12}

It helps in the conversion of homocysteine to methionine. Studies show vitamin B_{12} deficiency causes increase levels of urine methylmalonic acid levels in patients and worsens migraine. A possible mechanism of vitamin B_{12} action in migraine includes its excitatory role in the CNS by acting on NMDA receptors. It also plays a significant role in initiation, duration, and progression of migraine and activation of trigeminovascular system [71].

10.5 Feverfew

It is sold as capsules of dried leaves of the weed plant *Tanacetum parthenium*. Animal models show feverfew acts by inhibition of nitroglycerine-induced fos expression and inhibition of nuclear factor-kappa β. An open-label trial with *T. parthenium* (300 mg) plus *Salix alba* (white willow) for 12 weeks showed a decrease in pain intensity and duration of migraine. A randomized double-blind placebo-controlled trial (riboflavin 400 mg + magnesium 300 mg + feverfew 100 mg) for 3 months showed positive results. Recently two randomized clinical trials (RCT) of a purified stable extract of feverfew, MIG99, were ineffective in migraine, and clinical effects were very low with various complications [72].

10.6 Petasites (butterbur root)

Petasites hybridus is a potential poisonous plant but the detoxified root extract is safe. Mechanisms include inhibition of the synthesis of leukotrienes. It also decreases the intracellular concentration of calcium. It is used in the prophylaxis of migraine in children. A small study of 100 mg/day and a larger one of 150 mg/day vs placebo have shown efficacy [73].

11. Conclusion

With many newer agents now under clinical trials as well as in use, physicians should be aware of these drugs and their side effects, so they can use these agents for treating recurrent and chronic cases of migraine. Also, further well-designed clinical trials are needed to prove the efficacy of these agents in treatment of migraine. So, further research is needed to find out the safest and most effective treatment for chronic migraine, further designing proper animal models for studying migraine, to identify newer drug targets and how to prevent the migraine at the patient level from acute attack going in for chronic attack.

Conflict of interest

Nil.

Abbreviations

NSAIDS	nonsteroidal anti-inflammatory drugs
GJIC	gap junctional intercellular communication
CGRP	calcitonin gene-related peptide
NO	nitric oxide
NMDA	N-methyl-D-aspartate receptor
DHE	dihydroergotamine
ATP	adenosine triphosphate
ADP	adenosine diphosphate

Author details

Balaji Ommurugan[1*] and Vanishree Rao[2]

1 Quest Life Sciences Private Limited, India

2 Department of Pharmacology, MCOPS, Manipal, India

*Address all correspondence to: puntermmc@gmail.com

References

[1] Timothy et al. Impact of weather conditions on migraine in north eastern Nigeria. International Journal of Pharmacy and Pharmaceutical Sciences. 2011;**3**(3):133-136

[2] Vos T, Flaxman AD, Naghavi M, Lozano R, Michaud C, Ezzati M. Years lived with disability (YLDs) for 1160 sequelae of 289 diseases and injuries 1990-2010: A systematic analysis for the Global Burden of Disease Study 2010. Lancet. 2012;**380**(9859):2163-2196

[3] Natoli JL, Manack A, Dean B, Butler Q, Turkel CC, Stovner L, et al. Global prevalence of chronic migraine: A systematic review. Cephalalgia. 2009;**30**(5):599-609

[4] Abeer AK, Gihan SL. Flash dissolving sublingual almotriptan malate lyotabs for management of migraine. International Journal of Pharmacy and Pharmaceutical Sciences. 2017;**9**(1):125-131

[5] Headache Classification Subcommittee of the International Headache Society. The International Classification of Headache Disorders: 2nd edition. Cephalalgia. 2004;**24**(Suppl 1):9-160

[6] Lay CL, Broner SW. Migraine in women. Neurologic Clinics. 2009;**27**(2): 503-511

[7] Gilmore B, Michael M. Treatment of acute migraine headache. American Family Physician. 2011;**83**(3):271-280

[8] Simon RP, Greenberg DA, Aminoff MJ. Clinical Neurology. 7th ed. New York, NY: Lange Medical Books/ McGraw-Hill; 2009. pp. 85-88

[9] Gasparini C, Sutherland H, Griffiths L. Studies on the pathophysiology and genetic basis of migraine. Current Genomics. 2013;**14**(5):300

[10] Sarrouilhe D, Dejean C, Mesnil M. Involvement of gap junction channels in the pathophysiology of migraine with aura. Frontiers in Physiology. 2014;**5**:78

[11] Kaiser A, Russo A. CGRP and migraine: Could PACAP play a role too? Neuropeptides. 2013;**47**(6):451-461

[12] Kalra AA, Elliott D. Acute migraine: Current treatment and emerging therapies. Therapeutics and Clinical Risk Management. 2007;**3**(3):449

[13] Loder E. Triptan therapy in migraine. New England Journal of Medicine. 2010;**363**(1):63-70

[14] Lipton RB, Stewart WF, Stone AM, Láinez MJ, Sawyer JP. Stratified care vs step care strategies for migraine: The Disability in Strategies of Care (DISC) Study: A randomized trial. JAMA. 2000;**284**(20):2599-2605

[15] Study Group. Stratified care vs step care strategies for migraine: The Disability in Strategies of Care (DISC) Study: A randomized trial. JAMA. 2000;**284**(20):2599-2605

[16] Cady RK. Treating an acute attack of migraine. Headache. 2008;**48**(9): 1415-1416

[17] Hu XH, Ng-Mak D, Cady R. Does early migraine treatment shorten time to headache peak and reduce its severity? Headache. 2008;**48**(6):914-920

[18] Foley KA, Cady R, Martin V, et al. Treating early versus treating mild: Timing of migraine prescription medications among patients with diagnosed migraine. Headache. 2005;**45**(5):538-545

[19] Fox AW. Onset of effect of 5-HT1B/1D agonists: A model with pharmacokinetic validation. Headache. 2004;**44**(2):142-147

[20] Ferrari MD, Goadsby PJ, Roon KI, Lipton RB. Triptans (serotonin, 5-HT1B/1D agonists) in migraine: Detailed results and methods of a meta-analysis of 53 trials. Cephalalgia. 2002;**22**(8):633-658

[21] Shapiro RE, Tepper SJ. The serotonin syndrome, triptans, and the potential for drug-drug interactions. Headache. 2007;**47**(2):266-269

[22] Gillman K. Serotonin toxicity. Headache. 2008;**48**(4):640-641

[23] Baron EP, Tepper SJ. Revisiting the role of ergots in the treatment of migraine and headache. Headache. 2010;**50**(8):1353-1361

[24] Saper JR, Silberstein S. Pharmacology of dihydroergotamine and evidence for efficacy and safety in migraine. Headache. 2006;**46**(Suppl 4):171-181

[25] Klapper JA, Stanton J. Clinical experience with patient administered subcutaneous dihydroergotamine mesylate in refractory headaches. Headache. 1992;**32**(1):21-23

[26] Rabbie R, Derry S, Moore RA, McQuay HJ. Ibuprofen with or without an antiemetic for acute migraine headaches in adults. Cochrane Database of Systematic Reviews. 2010;**10**:CD008039

[27] Magis D, Schoenen J. Treatment of migraine: Update on new therapies. Current Opinion in Neurology. 2011;**24**(3):203-210

[28] Tfelt-Hansen P. Triptans vs other drugs for acute migraine. Are there differences in efficacy? A comment. Headache. 2008;**48**(4):601-605

[29] Lipton RB, Grosberg B, Singer RP, et al. Efficacy and tolerability of a new powdered formulation of diclofenac potassium for oral solution for the acute treatment of migraine: Results from the International Migraine Pain Assessment Clinical Trial (IMPACT). Cephalalgia. 2010;**30**(11):1336-1345

[30] Jones J, Sklar D, Dougherty J, White W. Randomized double-blind trial of intravenous prochlorperazine for the treatment of acute headache. JAMA. 1989;**261**(8):1174-1176

[31] Marmura MJ. Use of dopamine antagonists in treatment of migraine. Current Treatment Options in Neurology. 2012;**14**(1):27-35

[32] Kirthi V, Derry S, Moore RA, McQuay HJ. Aspirin with or without an antiemetic for acute migraine headaches in adults. Cochrane Database of Systematic Reviews. 2010;**4**:CD008041

[33] Bigal ME, Bordini CA, Speciali JG. Intravenous chlorpromazine in the emergency department treatment of migraines: A randomized controlled trial. Journal of Emergency Medicine. 2002;**23**(2):141-148

[34] Gallagher RM. Emergency treatment of intractable migraine. Headache. 1986;**26**:74-75

[35] Saper JR, Silberstein SD, Gordon CD, Hamel RL. Handbook of Headache Management. Baltimore: Williams & Wilkins; 1993. p. 49

[36] Krymchantowski AV, Barbosa JS. Dexamethasone decreases migraine recurrence observed after treatment with a triptan combined with a nonsteroidal anti-inflammatory drug. Arquivos de Neuro-psiquiatria. 2001;**59**(3B):708-711

[37] Hussain A, Young WB. Steroids and aseptic osteonecrosis (AON) in migraine patients. Headache. 2007;**47**(4):600-604

[38] Bigal ME, Lipton RB. Excessive acute migraine medication use and migraine progression. Neurology. 2008;**71**(22):1821-1828

[39] Loder E. Post-marketing experience with an opioid nasal spray for migraine: Lessons for the future. Cephalalgia. 2006;**26**(2):89-97

[40] Doods H, Arndt K, Rudolf K, Just S. CGRP antagonists: Unravelling the role of CGRP in migraine. Trends in Pharmacological Sciences. 2007;**28**(11):580-587

[41] Färkkilä M, Diener HC, Géraud G, Láinez M, Schoenen J, Harner N, et al. Efficacy and tolerability of lasmiditan, an oral 5-HT 1F receptor agonist, for the acute treatment of migraine: A phase 2 randomized, placebo-controlled, parallel-group, dose-ranging study. The Lancet Neurology. 2012;**11**(5):405-413

[42] Varty G, Grilli M, Forlani A, Fredduzzi S, Grzelak M, Guthrie D, et al. The antinociceptive and anxiolytic-like effects of the metabotropic glutamate receptor 5 (mgluR5) antagonists, MPEP and MTEP, and the mgluR1 antagonist, LY456236, in rodents: A comparison of efficacy and side-effect profiles. Psychopharmacology. 2005;**179**(1):207-217

[43] Giffin NJ, Kowacs F, Libri V, Williams P, Goadsby PJ, Kaube H. Effect of the adenosine A1 receptor agonist GR79236 on trigeminal nociception with blink reflex recordings in healthy human subjects. Cephalalgia. 2003;**23**(4):287-292

[44] Lassen LH, Ashina M, Christiansen I, Ulrich V, Grover R, Donaldson J, et al. Nitric oxide synthase inhibition: A new principle in the treatment of migraine attacks. Cephalalgia. 1998;**18**(1):27-32

[45] Tfelt H. Site of effect of LY2951742 for migraine prophylaxis. The Lancet Neurology. 2015;**14**(1):31-32

[46] Chabi A, Zhang Y, Jackson S, Cady R, Lines C, Herring WJ, et al. Randomized controlled trial of the orexin receptor antagonist Filorexant for migraine prophylaxis. Cephalalgia. 2015;**35**(5):379-388

[47] Meents J, Neeb RU. TRPV1 in migraine pathophysiology. Trends in Molecular Medicine. 2010;**16**(4):153-159

[48] Vogler B, Rapoport A, Tepper S, Sheftell F, Bigal M. Role of melatonin in the pathophysiology of migraine. CNS Drugs. 2006;**20**(5):343-350

[49] Magni G, Ceruti S. P2Y purinergic receptors: New targets for analgesic and antimigraine drugs. Biochemical Pharmacology. 2013;**85**(4):466-477

[50] Silberstein SD. Practice parameter: Evidence-based guidelines for migraine headache (an evidence-based review): Report of the Quality Standards Subcommittee of the American Academy of Neurology. Neurology. 2000;**55**(6):754-762

[51] Buchanan TM, Ramadan NM. Prophylactic pharmacotherapy for migraine headaches. Seminars in Neurology. 2006;**26**(2):188-198

[52] Bigal ME, Krymchantowski AV, Rapoport AM. Prophylactic migraine therapy: Emerging treatment options. Current Pain and Headache Reports. 2004;**8**:178-184

[53] Kaniecki RG. Migraine prevention with Carvedilol: A prospective, open-label trial. Headache. 2003;**43**:589

[54] Pietrobon D. Calcium channels and channelopathies of the central nervous system. Molecular Neurobiology. 2002;**25**:31-50

[55] Solomon GD. Verapamil in migraine prophylaxis-a five-year review. Headache: The Journal of Head and Face Pain. 1989;**29**(7):425-427

[56] Freitag FG, Collins SD, Carlson HA, et al. A randomized trial of divalproex sodium extended-release tablets in migraine prophylaxis. Neurology. 2002;**58**:1652-1659

[57] Shank RP, Gardocki JF, Streeter AJ, Maryanoff BE. An overview of the

preclinical aspects of topiramate: Pharmacology, pharmacokinetics, and mechanism of action. Epilepsia. 2000;**41**(Suppl 1):S3-S9

[58] Freitag FG, Diamond S, Diamond ML, et al. The prophylaxis of migraine with the GABA-agonist, tiagabine: A clinical report. Headache. 1999;**39**:354

[59] Vaisleb I, Neft R, Schor N. Role of Levetiracetam in prophylaxis of migraine headaches in childhood. Neurology. 2005;**64**:A343

[60] Krusz JC. Zonisamide in the treatment of headache disorders. Cephalalgia. 2001;**21**:374-375

[61] Ozyalcin SN, Talu GK, Kiziltan E, Yucel B, Ertas M, Disci R. The efficacy and safety of venlafaxine in the prophylaxis of migraine. Headache. 2005;**45**:144-152

[62] Schrader H, Stovner LJ, Helde G, Sand T, Bovim G. Prophylactic treatment of migraine with angiotensin converting enzyme inhibitor (lisinopril): Randomized, placebo controlled, crossover study. BMJ. 2001;**322**:19-22

[63] Tronvik E, Stovner LJ, Helde G, Sand T, Bovim G. Prophylactic treatment of migraine with an angiotensin II receptor blocker: A randomized controlled trial. JAMA. 2003;**289**:65-69

[64] Ashkenazi A, Silberstein AD. Botulinum toxin and other new approaches to migraine therapy. Annual Review of Medicine. 2004;**55**: 505-518

[65] Millán-Guerrero RO, Pineda-Lucatero AG, Hernández-Benjamín T, Tene CE, Pacheco MF. Nα-methylhistamine safety and efficacy in migraine prophylaxis: Phase I and phase II studies. Headache: The Journal of Head and Face Pain. 2003;**43**(4):389-394

[66] Hauge AW, Asghar MS, Schytz HW, Christensen K, Olesen J. Effects of tonabersat on migraine with aura: A randomized, double-blind, placebo-controlled crossover study. The Lancet Neurology. 2009;**8**(8):718-723

[67] Peikert A, Wilimzig C, Kohne-Volland R. Prophylaxis of migraine with oral magnesium: Results from a prospective, multi-center, placebo-controlled and double-blind randomized study. Cephalalgia. 1996;**16**:257-263

[68] Sandor PS, Di Clemente L, Coppola G, et al. Efficacy of coenzyme Q10 in migraine prophylaxis: A randomized controlled trial. Neurology. 2005;**64**:713-715

[69] Schoenen J, Jacquy J, Lenaerts M. Effectiveness of high-dose riboflavin in migraine prophylaxis: A randomized controlled trial. Neurology. 1998;**50**: 466-470

[70] Maizels M, Blumenfeld A, Burchette R. A combination of riboflavin, magnesium, and feverfew for migraine prophylaxis: A randomized trial. Headache. 2004;**44**:885-890

[71] Bianchi A, Salomone S, Caraci F, Pizza V, Bernardini R, D'Amato CC. Role of magnesium, coenzyme Q 10, riboflavin, and vitamin B 12 in migraine prophylaxis. Vitamins & Hormones. 2004;**69**:297-312

[72] Pittler MH, Ernst E. Feverfew for preventing migraine. Cochrane Database of Systematic Reviews. 2004;**1**: CD002286

[73] Lipton RB, Gobel H, Einhaupl KM, Wilks K, Mauskop A. Petasites hybridus root (butterbur) is an effective preventive treatment for migraine. Neurology. 2004;**63**:2240-2244

Chapter 3

Minimally Invasive Surgical Treatment of Migraine

Francesco Simonacci, Nicolò Bertozzi, Gianluigi Lago, Carlo Fante, Giuseppe Sanese and Edoardo Raposio

Abstract

Migraine headache (MH) is a very common disorder affecting 10–12% of the world's adult population. The first line therapy for migraine is usually a combination of conservative treatments but some patients seem to be refractory. For this group of patients, the minimally invasive surgical treatment of migraine might offer a solution. Migraine is usually caused by extracranial sensitive nerve compression due vascular, fascial or muscular structures nearby. The aim of migraine surgery is to relieve such compression at specific trigger points located in the occipital, temporal and frontal regions. From June 2011 until July 2019, we performed MH decompression surgeries in over 269 patients with either frontal, occipital, or temporal migraine trigger sites. In the occipital and temporal areas, nerve decompression was achieved by occipital and superficial temporal artery ligation, respectively. In patients suffering from frontal headache we performed both endoscopic nerve decompression and transpalpebral decompression. Among patient suffering from occipital migraine, 95% of them showed improvement of their condition, with 86% reporting complete relief. As concern temporal migraine, positive outcome was achieved in 83% of the patients (50% complete elimination and 33% partial improvement). In patient suffering from frontal migraine, positive results were observed in 94% of the patients (32% complete elimination, 62% partial improvement). Migraine is a common and debilitating condition that can be treated successfully with minimally invasive surgical procedure especially for those patients non-responding to medical therapies.

Keywords: migraine, tension-type headache, surgical therapy, minimally invasive surgery

1. Introduction

Migraine headache (MH) is known to affect over 324.1 million people worldwide [1, 2]. However, MH is still widely undiagnosed and undertreated. In US alone, MH treatment cost accounts for over $17 billion each year, without taking into consideration the indirect costs due to the 112 million annual workdays loss, which has an estimated cost of $14 billion [2–4]. Furthermore, MH has an even greater burden on patients' everyday life, their families, and the society.

Despite its prevalence and debilitating nature, MH is still widely undiagnosed and undertreated. A combination of pharmacologic (both abortive and preventive drugs) and non-pharmacological interventions (such as behavioral and lifestyle changes) are still the main treatment for MH patients. Nevertheless, most MH suffers remain refractory and does not achieve satisfactory relief.

Among the numerous hypotheses proposed over the years regarding MH etiology, none has come to clearly highlight its true nature. Some researchers have proposed that MH might be originated from a central neurovascular phenomenon, others have hypnotized a cortical neuronal hyperexcitability, others a cortical spreading depression, others an abnormal modulation of brain nociceptive system, and eventually others have demonstrated a central/peripheral activation with sensitization of the trigeminal system [2, 5]. But still MH pathophysiology is unclear and a matter of international debate.

Plastic surgeons were never looking for a surgical treatment for MH; however, this idea came into their eyes in 1999 following the reports made by patients that underwent corrugator supercilii muscle resection for forehead rejuvenation surgery and experienced elimination or improvement in their MH after [2, 5]. In 2000, Guyuron et al. [5] first reported in a retrospective study this association between corrugator supercilii muscle resection and disappearance or significant improvement in MH attacks, paving the way for a new MH origin and thus a new treatment option. Indeed MH appeared to be triggered by a peripheral activation of the trigeminal nerve, due to overstimulation of its branches (trigger points), followed by peripheral and central sensitization [5] And therefor, surgical decompression of these trigger sites might end up as an effective treatment modality of MH.

In the following years, independent researchers demonstrated the efficacy of botulin toxin injection for the treatment of MH [2]. These evidences supported the hypothesis that MH was determined by the peripheral activation of trigeminal nerve branches.

The trigger site was defined as the point where the MH attack starts and corresponds to the anatomical area of potential irritation of the trigeminal nerve branches [2, 6]. As a pathophysiological consequence of the chronic mechanical stimulation and irritation of the trigeminal nerve terminal branches, calcitonin gene-related peptide, substance P, and neurokinin are released [2, 5, 6]. These neuropeptides may cause the activation of the trigeminovascular system and the neurogenic inflammation leading to meningeal irritation, altered microvascular blood flow, central and peripheral trigeminal sensitization recognized as hyperalgesia, and cutaneous allodynia.

Eventually, multiple anatomical studies strengthened the trigger point theory of MH origin by demonstrating that musculature, vessels, bony foramen, and fascial bands could entrap or compress nerve branches at proposed migraine trigger sites [2, 6, 7].

Over the last 15 years, Guyuron conducted several studies providing foundation for this hypothesis and reported a reduction of the frequency, duration, and intensity of MH by at least half in 80–90% of patients [2, 5, 7–9]. In the same years, other independent groups reported similar findings by employing Guyuron's surgical approach, demonstrating the effectiveness of the procedure and the reproducibility of the results [2, 6]. However, the most striking evidence for the effectiveness of peripheral nerve decompression surgery for MH treatment came from a double-blind, sham-controlled study of Guyuron et al. [2, 8]. In this trial, 49 patients underwent decompressive surgery, while 26 underwent sham surgery. At least 50% reduction in MH was reported from 57.7% of patients of the sham surgery group and 83.7% in the actual surgery group ($p < 0.05$). Moreover, 57.1% of actual surgical group reported complete elimination of MH symptoms, compared with only 3.8% of patients in the sham surgery group ($p < 0.001$). At 1 year, all migraine headache measurements were significantly improved in the actual surgical group and were not influenced by the trigger site.

Following these studies, four were the main trigger sites identified:

1. I Trigger Site (Frontal): patients present with frontal symptoms; the glabellar muscles and/or supratrochlear and supraorbital vessels may irritate corresponding nerves.

2. II Trigger Site (Temporal): patients with temporal headaches; the temporalis muscle or the superficial temporal artery may cause inflammation of the zygomatic temporal branch of the trigeminal nerve (ZTN) or the auriculotemporal nerve (ATN).

3. III Trigger Site (Rhinogenic): patients complain of paranasal and retrobulbar headaches; deviated septum, contact between the turbinates and the septum, concha bullosa, septa bullosa, and other intranasal abnormalities may irritate the trigeminal end branches. This site will not be covered in the present chapter.

4. IV Trigger Site (Occipital): patients refer occipital symptoms: occipitalis, trapezius, and semispinalis capitis muscles, fascial bands, or the occipital artery can irritate the greater occipital nerve (GON) and/or the lesser occipital nerve (LON).

Following these evidences, it came to be clearly known that an essential step was detecting the precise site of pain onset (the trigger point) [2, 10–12]. Although patients might report diffuse headache, once they were asked to locate where the pain begins, they could precisely pinpoint it with one fingertip, and that was where the surgical treatment had to be performed in order to release the putative nerve branch. Surgeons' finger compression over the trigger point usually can evoke pain, thus confirming the exact location of trigger point. Nerve blocks and portable Doppler were also successfully investigated in order to confirm the trigger points and help less experienced surgeons, while preoperative botulinum toxin injections proved to be less useful. Lack or incomplete response should be carefully interpreted since it does not automatically exclude the suspected trigger point; indeed, incomplete release might have been performed. Careful analysis of patients' symptoms and meticulous physical examination can reliably guide the surgical planning. Indeed, MH origin and surgical deactivation procedures resembles closely upper limb compressing neuropathies. Therefore, surgical treatment for MH can successfully eliminate or reduce the MH frequency, intensity, and duration in a lasting manner, reducing the economic burden of MH sufferers, improving patients' performances and participation in daily life activities [2, 3–10]. But still, a percentage of patients are refractory to surgery [2, 7]. Possible explanations are that incomplete or incorrect detection of all of the trigger sites have occurred or that irritation sites are not correctly dealt by current surgical approaches [2, 6]. Rigorous patient screening and selection with proper identification of MH trigger points are mandatory for a successful surgical outcome; yet a thorough understanding of the anatomy is essential to ensure complete nerve release and prevent postoperative complications.

2. Surgical treatment

In order to be regarded eligible to undergo the surgery patients had to be diagnosed by a board-certified neurologist with: migraine without aura, tension-type headaches, or new daily persistent headaches with 4 or more attack each month for at least 6 months. Also, patients that do not benefit from any medications for their headache might undergo the procedure. However, patients with cluster headache, episodic tension-type headache, or secondary headaches are considered ineligible to undergo our procedure. Furthermore a CT scan or an MRI study must be performed prior to be regarded eligible for migraine deactivation surgery in order to rule out any cause of secondary migraine headache.

2.1 Frontal trigger site

The supraorbital nerve is a sensory nerve originating from the frontal branch of the ophthalmic division of the trigeminal nerve. In the majority of the cases, it passes through a supraorbital notch, which can be occasionally completed by a fibrous band. Here the nerve displays an intimate relationship with the corrugator supercilii muscle. The reason why some patients do not respond to the surgical decompression of the only supraorbital nerve and need a more medial muscular resection is that the supratrochlear nerve may be involved [2, 13–16]. The supratrochlear nerve is the smallest terminal branch of the frontal nerve, which itself originates from the ophthalmic division of the trigeminal nerve. It emerges between the trochlea and the supraorbital foramen. Another source of compression can be the interaction of nerves with the vascular structures. The main vessels that may be involved are the supratrochlear and the supraorbital arteries.

Patients who suffered from frontal migraine headache can be treated with either endoscopic or transpalpebral approach. In our experience, we performed both procedures to decompress supraorbital and supratrochlear nerves [13–16]. However, endoscopic nerve decompression cannot be performed on patients with long foreheads (8 cm measured from the anterior hairline to the supraorbital ridge) or on patients with significant curvature to the forehead, as endoscopic access would have been difficult to impossible. In our experience, endoscopic approach did not allow to treat the vascular compression of supraorbital and supratrochlear nerves by corresponding ectasic arteries [2, 13–16]. Transpalpebral approach for frontal trigger site deactivation was performed by means a supratarsal crease incision involving up to two-thirds of the medial limit of the caudal portion of the conventional upper blepharoplasty incision. The upper eyelid, glabellar area, and the lower forehead were infiltrated with local anesthesia composed by 40-cc Carbocaine 1% + 40-cc NaCl 0.9% and 20-cc sodium bicarbonate 8.4%. After raising a skin-orbicularis oculi muscle flap above the level of the septum, the orbicularis muscle was dissected in a cephalic direction. The dissection was continued to the supraoribtal rim. The corrugator supercilii muscle protecting the supraorbital and supratrochlear nerves was elevated and by dissection the exposure of depressor supercilii muscle was performed. After selective myotomy of depressor and corrugator supercilii muscles, the lateral fibers of the procerus muscle encasing the supratrochlear nerve were dissected. Once the supraorbital and supratrochlear nerves were isolated, they were decompressed by the cauterization of the concomitant ectasic arteries. The cutaneous access was closed with absorbable sutures, and steri-strips were positioned at level of superior eyelids bilaterally. The endoscopic selective myotomies technique was performed with a single access by mean a specifically modified endoscope (Karl Storz, Tuttlingen, Germany). With the patient supine and the head in a neutral position, frontal trigger nerves were located. Skin markings were drawn above the eyebrow bilaterally, at the mid-pupillary line (supraorbital nerve) and 1 cm medially (supratrochlear nerve). Local anesthesia with diluted 40-cc Carbocaine 1% + 40-cc NaCl 0.9% and 20-cc sodium bicarbonate 8.4% was injected in the forehead, between the glabellar region and about 2 cm behind the anterior hairline. A single 1.5-cm incision was then performed on the midline, 1 cm behind the frontal hairline. All tissues were dissected until the periosteum layer. The lateral anatomic limit of the undermined area was the temporal region, bilaterally. In order to lift the frontal skin during the endoscopic procedure (and better visualize the anatomic structures) nylon 1-0 sutures were placed in the superciliary region at each side of both supratrochlear and supraorbital nerves bilaterally. Our modified endoscope (Karl Storz, Tuttlingen, Germany) consists of a 9-mm trocar with an air/insufflator/suction triple valve, a straight Hopkins telescope with fiber-light transmission, a Wittmöser operating sheath with a connection for high-frequency diathermy, and a specifically designed elliptical-tipped wire loop electrode for electrocautery. The modified endoscope was inserted through the incision in the subgaleal plane and used to perform endoscopically assisted section of the corrugator supercilii, depressor supercilii, and procerus muscles bilaterally, with the purpose of decompressing the supraorbital and supratrochlear nerves bilaterally. At the end of the procedure, after an accurate hemostasis, the cutaneous access was closed with absorbable suture, without any drainage; a compressive bandage was positioned all around undermined region [2, 13–16] (**Figure 1**).

2.2 Temporal trigger site

The ATN and ZTN are the two primary trigger points in the temporal migraine. The ATN is one of the terminal braches of the mandibular (V1) division of the trigeminal nerve. The ZTN is one of the terminal braches of the maxillary division (V2) of the trigeminal nerve [17–21].

It is our experience that the ATN is more often involved than the ZTN as temporal MH trigger given the close relationship with the superficial temporal artery (STA). Therefore, our surgical procedure primarily aims at eliminating the pulsatile irritation of the STA to the ATN by ligating the artery prior to and above the intersection or coiling segment. However, we perform ZTN decompression whenever STA-ATN relationship is not intraoperatively observed.

We perform both our personal decompression techniques under local assisted anesthesia [17].

For ATN decompression surgery, we usually marked a 1.5-cm incision where patients pinpoint the painful spot above the insertion of auricular helix at level of temporal area. A handheld Doppler was regularly used to locate the STA, since we

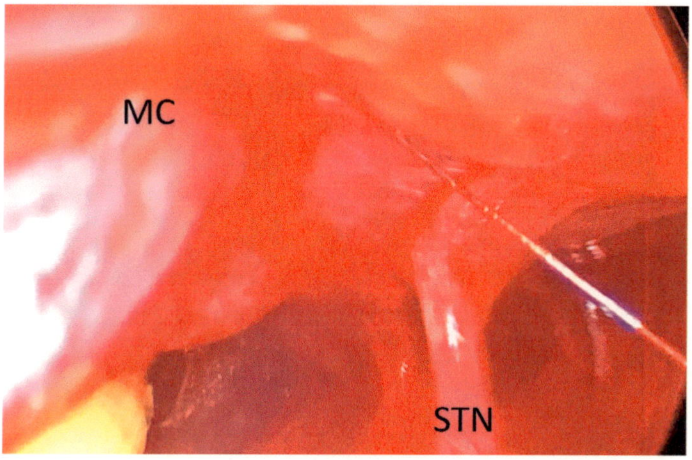

Figure 1.
Endoscopic selective myotomies of corrugator supercilii muscle (MC) with decompression of supratrochlear nerve (STN).

observed 100% correlation rate between the trigger point identified and a close ATN-STA relationship (being either a simple crossover or a helical intertwining). Once the incision was made, dissection was taken with the help of blunt tipped scissors to expose and isolate both ATN and STA, which was ligated both proximally and caudally to the area of nerve-artery intersection [17].

When it was necessary to decompress the ZTN, we made 3-cm cutaneous incision 8–10 mm behind the temporal hairline and took dissection deep to the deep temporal fascia by the blunt tip scissors. We opened the inferior temporal septum exposing the inferior temporal compartment that contains the ZTN, sentinel vessels, and temporal branches of facial nerve (that must be carefully preserved by incorporating it in the roof of the elevated flap). Then we widened the exit of the ZTN through temporal muscle and fascia, and the sentinel vessels were cauterized only when patients described a pulsating pain in the temporal region [17] (**Figure 2**).

2.3 Occipital trigger site

The common occipital headache symptoms here can be caused by the compression of the greater, lesser, and third occipital nerves. This is due to the presence of muscular and fascial entrapments and also because of their interaction with the vascular structures [2, 4, 7, 22]. The greater occipital nerve originates from the medial branch of the C2 dorsal root. It curves to reach the occipital region, running caudal to the inferior oblique muscle and sometimes piercing it. Then it reaches the semispinalis muscle, where it is possible to identify the deepest potential compression point of the nerve. The course of the nerve in the area of the superior nuchal

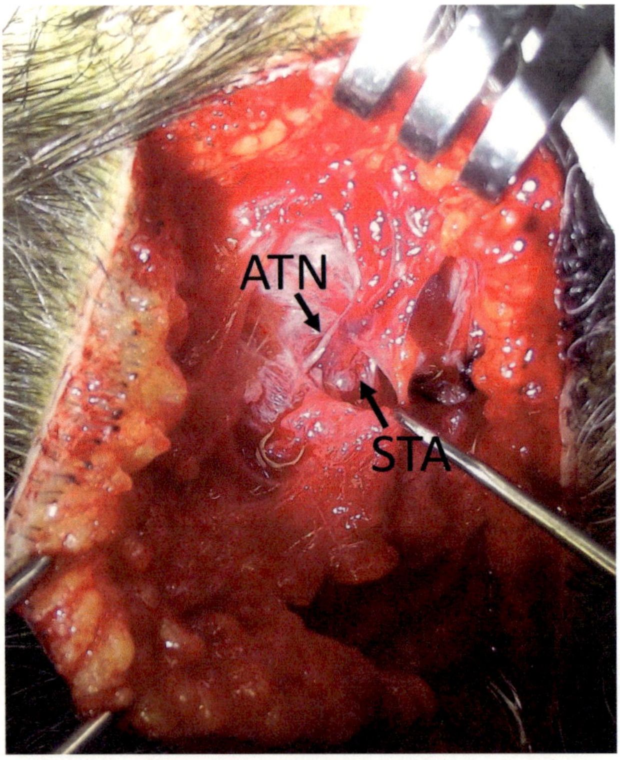

Figure 2.
Close auriculotemporal nerve (ATN) and superficial temporal artery (STA) relationship.

line is variously described, because of the large anatomical variability that these structures present. The latest studies have shown the exact location of the intramuscular course of the nerve: it is located 3 cm below and 1.5 cm lateral to the occipital protuberance [2, 4, 7, 22]. Possible trigger points can be found at its entrance into the deep fascia underlying the semispinalis or the muscle itself or at level of the entrance of the nerve in the semispinalis capitis and trapezius muscles. Other possible compression is where the nerve pierces the tendinous insertion of the trapezius into the nuchal line [2, 4, 7, 22].

Because of the surgical decompression of the nerve, the semispinalis capitis and the trapezius together with the splenius and the occipital muscles are resected with multiple myotomies.

However, based on our study, the close relationship found between the great occipital nerve and the occipital artery in the region of the superior nuchal line is the principal trigger point of occipital migraine.

This artery is the main vessel running through the occipital area. It arises from the external carotid artery, and it runs medially to the mastoid process on the temporal bone. It then reaches the occipital region, boring the deep cervical fascia between the sternocleidomastoid and the cranial attachment of the trapezius. At this point it can be found in the subcutaneous layer leaving many convoluted branches and anastomosing with the contralateral artery [3]. In more than 50% of the cases, an intimate anatomical relationship was found. There are two possible types of interaction: they can coil together (70%) or the other possibility is a simple crossing (30%) with the nerve passing superficial to the artery [2, 4, 7, 22].

Furthermore, minor trigger sites are also described in this area [2, 4, 7, 22]. It is related to the lesser occipital nerves, which can be similarly compressed by fascial bands and the occipital artery branches. If the lesser occipital nerve is affected, it can be responsible of laterally located pain symptoms. It arises from C2 or rarely from C3 dorsal root; it emerges from the posterior border of the sternocleidomastoids, seldom piercing it, and then ascends along it. The emergence point was found with a 3-cm diameter located 6.5 cm from midline and 5.3 cm below the line drawn between the two external auditory canals.

Surgical treatment of occipital trigger site aims at removing the potential compression points of the greater and the lesser occipital nerve along their course throughout the semispinalis, the splenius and the trapezius muscles to the subcutaneous tissue of the occipital scalp. The avulsion of the third occipital nerve (TON) during the occipital migraine surgery does not improve clinical outcomes. According to Guyuron et al. [7], Lin et al. [23], Dash et al. [24], and Lee et al. [25], the currently adopted procedure for treatment of the occipital trigger site, undertaken under general anesthesia, relies first on an incision in the occipital scalp and extensive undermining through which a small portion of the semispinalis capitis muscle is removed. This muscle is usually pierced by the greater occipital nerve (GON), lesser occipital nerves (LON) bilaterally. Subsequently, a subcutaneous flap is transposed between the GON and the muscle to avoid nerve impingement [7, 23–25].

As regards our experience [26–28], we performed the occipital decompression surgical technique with the patient prone, under local assisted anesthesia. After injecting 40-cc of diluted Carbocaine 1% + 40-cc NaCl 0.9% and 20-cc sodium bicarbonate 8.4%, two horizontal occipital scalp incisions 5 cm in length were performed along the superior nuchal line bilaterally, at the location of arterial signal detected preoperatively by portable Doppler. Underneath the subcutaneous tissue, an accurate dissection of occipital, trapezius, splenius capitis and semispinalis capitis muscles allowed to identify the GON and vascular bundle (occipital

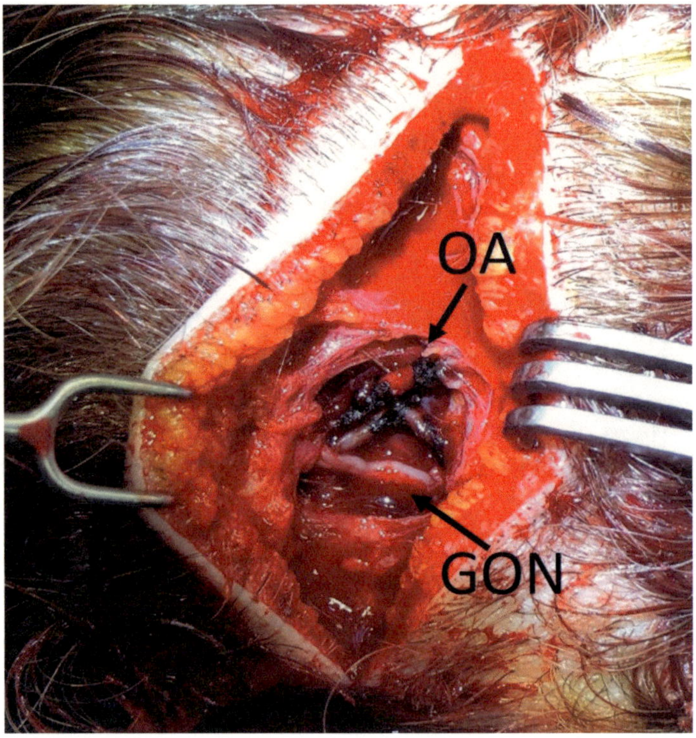

Figure 3.
Cauterization of ectasic occipital artery (OA) with decompression of greater occipital nerve (GON).

artery). When we found a dilated (or frankly aneurysmatic) occipital artery in close connection with the GON, we ligated or cauterized the vessel without any other surgical maneuvers except for accurate hemostasis and skin closure.

In the remaining cases in which vascular compression was not found we adopted a more conventional approach based on neurolysis of the GON and LON by undermining the occipital, trapezius, splenius capitis and semispinalis capitis muscles and following the nerve course caudally as possible [26, 27]. At the end of the procedure, after an accurate hemostasis, the cutaneous access was sutured with absorbable threads, without any drainage. No trichotomy was needed, and the scar from the incision was hidden in the patient's hair. The total operative time was no longer than 90 min for bilateral incisions, but often it was less than 60 minutes when the relevant anatomical structures were easily identified [27, 28] (**Figure 3**).

3. Results

From June 2011 until July 2019, we performed MH decompression surgeries in over 269 patients with either frontal, occipital, or temporal migraine trigger sites [2, 13–17, 26–28].

As concern the frontal migraine we performed 72 decompression surgeries (65 bilateral and 7 unilateral). After a mean follow-up of 24 months (range: 12–97 months), patients with frontal trigger site migraine reported a 94% positive response to surgery (32% complete relief and 62% significant improvement), while 6% had no change in their symptoms. Among total patients underwent MH frontal decompression surgeries, 24 patients (34.2%) experienced secondary trigger point emergence following primary occipital and/or temporal migraine surgery.

Among these, 20 patients had two trigger points (18 frontal and occipital, 2 frontal and temporal) while 4 patients had all three trigger points. All patients continue to experience a quality of life better than before surgery, and all would have the surgery again. The learning curve and the experience of the operator play also an important role when evaluating clinical outcomes (**Figure 4**).

Decompression surgeries to treat temporal trigger point were 56. Among these, 53 had monolateral localization, while 3 had bilateral one. Because the ATN-STA close relationship was observed intraoperatively in 47 surgeries the only ATN decompressions were performed. Whereas ZTN deactivation procedures were performed during the same operative session 6 times, since no ATN-STA close relationship was encountered. Therefore, we observed ATN-STA close relationship in 85.3% of patients; single STA-ATN intersection accounted for 83.7% of the cases, while helical intertwining accounted for 16.3%. After a mean follow-up of 24 months (range, 3–67 months), patients complaining for temporal MH had 83% positive surgical outcome (50% complete MH elimination, 33% significant improvement). Among total MH temporal decompression surgeries, 29 patients (49%) experienced secondary or tertiary trigger point emergence following primary migraine surgery. Among these 22 had two trigger points (20 temporal and occipital, 2 frontal and occipital) while 4 patients had all three trigger points (**Figure 5**).

As concern occipital migraine we performed 141 decompression surgeries (94 bilateral and 47 unilateral). In 119 patients with occipital migraine, we found a dilated occipital artery in close connection with the GON and we ligated the vessel without any other surgical maneuvers. In 22 patients with occipital migraine, vascular compression was not found and we adopted a conventional approach based on neurolysis of the GON and LON from muscles. We gathered data from questionnaires completed before and after surgery. After a mean follow up of 24 months (range: 3–67 months), patients with occipital migraine had positive response in 94.9% (86.8% complete relief and 8.1% significant improvement), and 5.1% did not get any better. As for the 119 patients who underwent dilated occipital artery ligation, positive response 95.5% (90% complete relief and 5.5% significant improvement) and 4.5% did not get any better. As for the 22 patients who did not undergo occipital artery ligation, we observed positive response in 91% (76% complete relief and 15% significant improvement) of the subjects while 9% did not get any better. All the patients without improvement of the symptoms after occipital artery ligation (3.5%) suffered of unilateral occipital migraine and referred complete relief after contralateral secondary surgery. Total patients underwent MH decompression

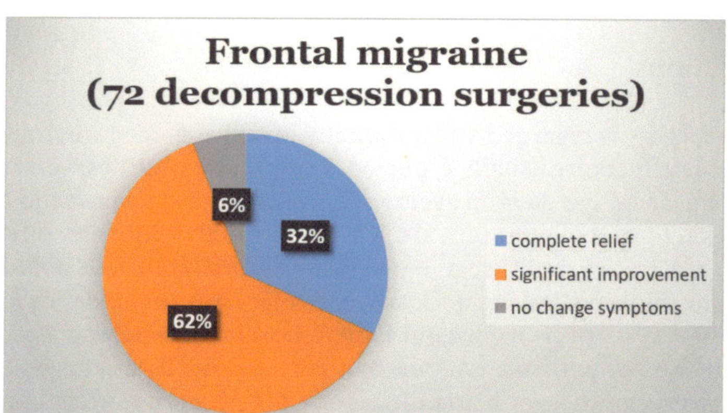

Figure 4.
Results of fontal migraine decompression surgeries from June 2011 until July 2019.

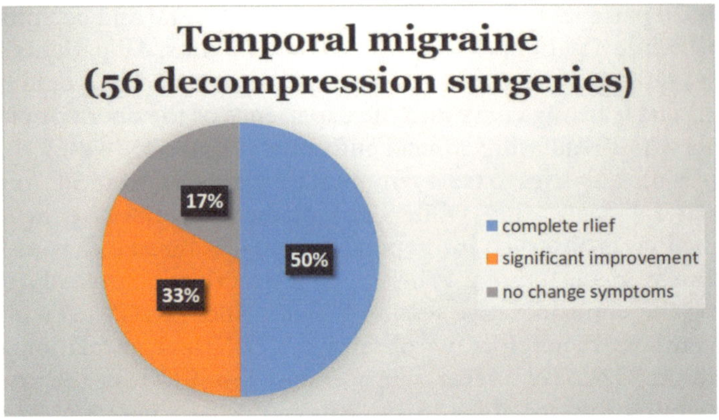

Figure 5.
Results of temporal migraine decompression surgeries from June 2011 until July 2019.

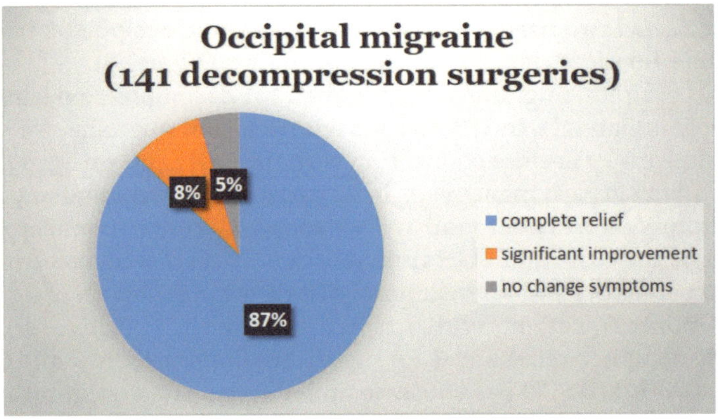

Figure 6.
Results of occipital migraine decompression surgeries from June 2011 until July 2019.

surgeries, 42 patients (29.7%) experienced secondary or tertiary trigger point emergence following primary migraine surgery. Among these, 38 patients had two trigger points (18 occipital and frontal, 20 occipital and temporal) while 4 patients had all three trigger points (**Figure 6**).

4. Complications

Migraine surgery is regarded as a minimally invasive procedure; thus, no concerning side effects are usually reported. Temporary anesthesia occurred in all patients, which lasted 163 days on average [2, 13–17, 26–29]. Minor and transient complications reported in literature are lasting occipital numbness, intense itching after surgery, hypertrophic scar, incisional cellulitis, transient mild incisional alopecia or hair thinning, lasting neck stiffness that have an incidence ranging from 1 to 5% [2, 13–17, 26–29]. As regard our experience, intense itching after surgery was present in 30% of patients, temporary anesthesia in all patients while postoperative infections, seromas, or hematomas were not observed. All patients that were refractory to surgery did not report worsening in their MH at any follow-up. As concern frontal migraine decompression surgeries all patients experienced frontal and/or upper eyelid edema of various degrees. Usually the edema resolves by the fifth postoperative day. Ecchymosis of both upper and lower eyelids follows surgery. No treatment needed to be given as these collateral events resolve by themselves; boric water applications three times a day helped the process of reabsorption of the edema. As previously stated, the only hypothetical serious complication that might occur within the 12 h following the surgery is the compression of the optical nerve due to the descent of the edema into the posterior orbicular space. In these cases, prompt recognition of patient's sight modification is mandatory in order to urgently decompress the optic nerve. Patients with particularly thin skin of the frontal region may develop postoperative burn-like scar because of the endoscopic electrocautery. The most common complication after site temporal migraine surgeries is slight hollowing of the temple (54% incidence rate). Nerve avulsion might be associated with neuroma formation, although it is not reported in literature of any neuroma following avulsion of ATN and/or ZTN [2, 13–17, 26–28].

Based on our data collected, secondary trigger point emergence following primary occipital migraine surgery occurred in 35% of patients. However, we routinely deactivate the main trigger site first, and then a second or third surgery is performed at the remaining sites 3 months after each surgery. MH recurrence may occur from 1 up to 3 months after surgery; thus the result may be regarded as permanent only after the third postoperative month [2, 13–17, 26–28].

Conflict of interest

The authors declare no conflict of interest.

Author details

Francesco Simonacci[1*], Nicolò Bertozzi[1], Gianluigi Lago[1], Carlo Fante[1], Giuseppe Sanese[2] and Edoardo Raposio[1]

1 Department of Medicine and Surgery, Plastic Surgery Unit, University of Parma, Parma, Italy

2 Division of Plastic and Reconstructive Surgery, University "Tor Vergata", Rome, Italy

*Address all correspondence to: francescosimonacci@hotmail.it

References

[1] World Health Organization. The Global Burden of Disease, 2004 Update. Geneva, Switzerland: World Health Organization; 2004

[2] Raposio E, Bertozzi N, Bordin C, Simonacci F. Surgical therapy of migraine and tension-type headaches. In: Turker H, editor. Current Perspectives on Less-Known Aspects of Headache. Zagreb, Croatia: InTech; 2017. pp. 93-114

[3] Faber C, Garcia RM, Davis J, Guyuron B. A socioeconomic analysis of surgical treatment of migraine headaches. Plastic and Reconstructive Surgery. 2012;**129**:871-877

[4] Chmielewski L, Liu MT, Guyuron B. The role of occipital artery resection in the surgical treatment of occipital migraine headaches. Plastic and Reconstructive Surgery. 2013;**131**:351e-356e

[5] Guyuron B, Varghai A, Michelow BJ, Thomas T, Davis J. Corrugator supercilii muscle resection and migraine headaches. Plastic and Reconstructive Surgery. 2000;**106**:429-437

[6] Janis JE, Barker JC, Javadi C, Ducic I, Hagan R, Guyuron B. A review of current evidence in the surgical treatment of migraine headaches. Plastic and Reconstructive Surgery. 2014;**134**:131-141

[7] Guyuron B, Kriegler JS, Davis J, Amini SB. Comprehensive surgical treatment of migraine headaches. Plastic and Reconstructive Surgery. 2005;**115**(1):1-9

[8] Guyuron B, Reed D, Kriegler JS, Davis J, Pashmini N, Amini S. A placebo-controlled surgical trial of the treatment of migraine headaches. Plastic and Reconstructive Surgery. 2009;**124**:461-468

[9] Guyuron B, Kriegler JS, Davis J, Amini SB. Five-year outcome of surgical treatment of migraine headaches. Plastic and Reconstructive Surgery. 2011;**127**:603-608

[10] Punjabi A, Brown M, Guyuron B. Emergence of secondary trigger sites after primary migraine surgery. Plastic and Reconstructive Surgery. 2016;**137**:712e-716e

[11] Guyuron B, Nahabet E, Khansa I, Reed D, Janis JE. The current means for detection of migraine headache trigger sites. Plastic and Reconstructive Surgery. 2015;**136**:860-867

[12] Liu MT, Armijo BS, Guyuron B. A comparison of outcome of surgical treatment of migraine headaches using a constellation of symptoms versus botulinum toxin type A to identify the trigger sites. Plastic and Reconstructive Surgery. 2012;**129**:413-419

[13] Raposio E, Caruana G. Frontal endoscopic myotomies for chronic headache. The Journal of Craniofacial Surgery. 2015;**26**:e201-e203

[14] Raposio E, Caruana G. Minimally invasive endoscopic surgical treatment of headache. In: Raposio E, editor. Atlas of Endoscopic Plastic Surgery. New York, N.Y: Springer; 2016. pp. 17-21

[15] Caruana G, Bertozzi N, Boschi E, Grieco MP, Grignaffini E, Raposio E. Endoscopic forehead surgery for migraine therapy personal technique. Annali Italiani di Chirurgia. 2014;**85**:583-586

[16] Caruana G, Grignaffini E, Raposio E. Endoscopic forehead muscle resection for nerve decompression: A modified procedure. Plastic and Reconstructive Surgery. Global Open. 2015;**3**:e342

[17] Bertozzi N, Simonacci F, Lago G, Bordin C, Raposio E. Surgical therapy of temporal triggered migraine headache. Plastic and Reconstructive Surgery. Global Open. 2018;**6**:e1980

[18] Chim H, Okada HC, Brown MS, et al. The auriculotemporal nerve in etiology of migraine headaches: Compression points and anatomical variations. Plastic and Reconstructive Surgery. 2012;**130**:336-341

[19] Janis JE, Hatef DA, Ducic I, et al. Anatomy of the auriculotemporal nerve: Variations in its relationship to the superficial temporal artery and implications for the treatment of migraine headaches. Plastic and Reconstructive Surgery. 2010;**125**:1422-1428

[20] Janis JE, Hatef DA, Thakar H, et al. The zygomaticotemporal branch of the trigeminal nerve: Part II. Anatomical variations. Plastic and Reconstructive Surgery. 2010;**126**:435-442

[21] Iwanaga J, Watanabe K, Saga T, et al. Anatomical study of the superficial temporal branches of the auriculotemporal nerve: Application to surgery and other invasive treatments to the temporal region. Journal of Plastic, Reconstructive & Aesthetic Surgery. 2017;**70**:370-374

[22] Gfrerer L, Raposio E, Ortiz R, Austen WG Jr. Surgical treatment of migraine headache: Back to the future. Plastic and Reconstructive Surgery. 2018;**142**:1036-1045

[23] Lin SH, Lin HC, Jeng CH, Hsieh CH, Lin YH, Chen CC. Experience of surgical treatment for occipital migraine in Taiwan. Annals of Plastic Surgery. 2016;**76**:S80-S84

[24] Dash KS, Janis JE, Guyuron B. The lesser and third occipital nerves and migraine headaches. Plastic and Reconstructive Surgery. 2005;**115**:1752-1758

[25] Lee M, Lineberry K, Reed D, Guyuron B. The role of the third occipital nerve in surgical treatment of occipital migraine headaches. Journal of Plastic, Reconstructive & Aesthetic Surgery. 2013;**66**:1335-1339

[26] Polotto S, Simonacci F, Grignaffini E, Grieco MP, Raposio E. Surgical treatment of frontal and occipital migraines: A comparison of results. Plastic and Reconstructive Surgery. Global Open. 2016;**4**:e653

[27] Raposio E, Caruana G. Tips for the surgical treatment of occipital nerve-triggered headaches. European Journal of Plastic Surgery. 2017;**40**:177-182

[28] Raposio E, Simonacci F, Bertozzi N, Bellini E. Occipital migraine: A vascular approach. Plastic and Reconstructive Surgery. Global Open. 2017;**5**:78

[29] Ducic I, Hartmann EC, Larson EE. Indications and outcomes for surgical treatment of patients with chronic migraine headaches caused by occipital neuralgia. Plastic and Reconstructive Surgery. 2009;**123**:1453-1461

Chapter 4

Therapeutic Management: When and What

Theodoros Mavridis, Marianthi Breza, Christina I. Deligianni and Dimos D. Mitsikostas

Abstract

Migraine is a widespread brain disease that is classified as the second most disabling condition and has the third highest prevalence of all medical conditions. Despite its non-emergent or life-threatening nature, migraine can progress to chronic type, a subform associated with significant morbidity and drug overuse. In the management of migraine, it is important therefore to introduce early prophylactic treatment in order to limit migraine chronification. In this chapter, we will go through all the treatment options, both acute and preventive, pharmaceutical and non-pharmaceutical following this flowchart: 1. Introduction; 2. General principles; 2.1 Symptomatic therapy; 2.2 Prophylactic management; 3. Pharmaceutical therapies; 3.1 Symptomatic; 3.1.1 Disease-specific; 3.1.2 No disease-specific; 3.2 Prophylactic; 3.2.1 Disease-specific; 3.2.2 No disease-specific; 3.3 Non-Pharmaceutical therapies; 3.4 Neuromodulation; 3.4.1 Invasive; 3.4.5 Non-invasive; 3.5 Nutrient (nutraceuticals); 3.6 Dietary interventions; 3.7 Acupuncture; 3.8 Physical therapy; 4. Cognitive behavioral therapies; 5. Patient centricity and patient education.

Keywords: therapy, pharmaceutical therapy, non-pharmaceutical therapy, symptomatic treatment, prophylactic treatment, devices, cognitive behavioral therapy, physical therapy, acupuncture, nutrient, nutraceuticals, dietary interventions, patient centricity, patient

1. Introduction

The last decade heralded a new era in migraine therapeutics, with the emergence of novel targeted therapies. Recent advances in the field of migraine research have resulted to newly available acute and preventive treatment options, including gepants (calcitonin gene-related peptide (CGRP)-receptor antagonists), anti-CGRP/R monoclonal antibodies (mAbs), and ditans (5-HT_{1F} receptor agonists). Several advances were also achieved in non-pharmaceutical therapeutics, with the advent of devices for vagus nerve stimulation (VNS), external trigeminal nerve stimulation (eTNS), and transcranial magnetic stimulation (TMS) [1]. This chapter provides a comprehensive overview of available therapeutic approaches in migraine (pharmaceutical and non-pharmaceutical), summarizing both acute and prophylactic options.

The therapeutic management of migraine is multidisciplinary, including both pharmaceutical and non-pharmaceutical approaches. The choice of pharmaceutical treatment should be individualized, taking into consideration the characteristics of the migraine attack, the patients' comorbidities, and treatment preferences [2, 3].

The symptomatic migraine treatment aims to rapidly relief headache, restore function, and prevent recurrence. To date, simple analgesics, nonsteroidal anti-inflammatory drugs (NSAIDs), and triptans are the most widely prescribed medications for acute migraine [1]. Triptans (selective serotonin 5-$HT_{1B/1D}$ receptor agonists) have shown to inhibit the release of calcitonin gene-related peptide (CGRP) and were first approved for acute migraine therapy in the early 1990s [4]. However, these drugs are not efficient in all patients and might have vasoconstrictive properties that could be a contraindication [1], leaving room for new, disease-specific symptomatic treatments. The development of two novel classes of drugs, gepants (CGRP receptor antagonists) and ditans (serotonin 5-HT1F receptor agonists), for the symptomatic treatment of acute migraine allows management of patients that do not tolerate or respond to the above agents [1].

Every year about 3% of patients convert from episodic to chronic migraine (≥15 headache days per month, of which ≥8 migraine days) [1]. It is important therefore to introduce early prophylactic treatment in order to limit migraine chronification. The calcitonin gene-related peptide (CGRP) antagonists were approved in 2018 and represent the first class of novel targeted medications specifically designed and approved for migraine prevention. The newly approved monoclonal antibodies against the ligand CGRP or its receptor (anti-CGRP/R mAbs) are fremanezumab, erenumab, and galcanezumab, while eptinezumab is waiting for approval in 2020 [5]. Ubrogepant, lasmiditan, and rimegepant are emerging acute migraine therapies that are also waiting to be added to the arsenal of current migraine management [6].

The use of non-pharmaceutical approaches is recommended as adjunct therapy or as alternative to the first-line pharmaceutical treatment [7, 8]. Complementary interventions are used to minimize the overuse of acute pain medication or adverse effects (AEs) and as alternative when preventive pharmaceutical therapy fails or is contraindicated. Non-pharmaceutical strategies suggested include approved devices for migraine, cognitive behavioral therapies, physical therapy, improving quality of sleep, acupuncture, and dietary solutions [9–11].

Overall, novel therapies signify a paradigm shift in migraine management and not only bring new hope to patients suffering for migraine but also change the clinician's approach to the treatment of migraine [1]. While migraine therapy is currently undergoing tremendous development, unmet needs of patients remain, which, if addressed, have the potential to further enhance available treatment options and improve the quality of life of migraineurs. Identification of predictive biomarkers for responders and nonresponders to therapies, and elucidation of underlying migraine pathophysiology are still lacking, and are essential for the development of novel therapeutic targets and individualized migraine prevention.

2. General principles

To date, there is no cure for migraine, but migraine can be successfully treated in many cases.

Therefore, education of patients is of great significance. This could be achieved by thoroughly explaining patients' disorder, purpose, and means of management. Patient information leaflets on migraine and management are available from the Headache Federations (Lifting The Burden) [12]. Prior to treatment and during follow-up assessments, patients should be monitored and evaluated using recommended assessment tools: the HALT-30 Index that assesses burden in terms of lost productive time, the Migraine Disability Assessment Test (MIDAS), the Headache

Impact Test (HIT-6), which evaluates the headache impact and severity, and the Headache Under-Response to Treatment Questionnaire (HURT), which evaluates efficacy and ensures that the optimal treatment has been reached [12–18]. A calendar is recommended to be used by the patients with migraine, in order to monitor acute medication or overuse [12].

Regarding triggers and predisposing factors, modification of lifestyle, where applicable, is recommended. However, triggers are not always avoidable. Over the years, the significance of trigger factors in migraine has been overemphasized [2, 12].

Management of migraine in special populations (pregnant women, children, nonresponders, and elderly with comorbidities) should be carried out only by headache specialists [12].

The purpose of pharmacotherapy of primary headache is mostly to control symptoms in order to minimize the impact of the disorder on each individual patient's life and lifestyle. For treatment to be effective, first, it is crucial that the correct diagnosis has been made. Then, the choice of therapy requires an individual approach, as each patient is unique. Severity and frequency of attacks, disability causing, other symptoms, time to peak, patient preferences, comorbidities, drug interactions, side effects, and prior therapies that failed should be all taken into consideration [2].

Acute treatment should be taken as early as possible in the headache phase to abort an attack. Prophylactic treatment is administered periodically in order to reduce the frequency and severity of migraine attacks. Often a combination of acute and prophylactic treatment is needed [2].

Pharmaceutical treatment for acute attacks is used almost by all patients with migraine. Prophylactic treatment should be recommended in nonresponders to acute treatment or not well-controlled patients, whose quality of life is impaired by migraine [12].

The following recommendations are highlighted from the Headache Consortiums and Federations Management principles, as the main clinical recommendations that should be prioritized in pharmaceutical treatment.

2.1 Symptomatic therapy

When migraine attacks are not severe or disabling for less than 4 days per month, only symptomatic therapy is considered [2]. It is important to know when to treat a migraine attack and which therapy and route of administration are preferred, especially in patients experiencing nausea and vomiting. Generally, patients are advised to receive the abortive treatment as early as possible in the attack to reduce the intensity and duration of migraine as well as the accompanying features. In case of an inadequate response, it can be repeated after two hours (same or other treatment). There is a restriction on the duration of usage of symptomatic treatment due to the probability of developing medication overuse headache (MOH). Thus, taking into account the criteria of ICHD-III [19], intake of symptomatic treatment should not exceed 10 days per month for ergotamine, triptans, or combinations of drugs, or 15 days per month for NSAIDs, paracetamol, and aspirin.

Non-opioid analgesics (eg. NSAIDs, aspirin and paracetamol, or combinations with caffeine) with the addition of antiemetics (if needed), are the first-line treatment for mild to moderate attacks. Analgesics should be administered early in the attack and in adequate dosage, and during the aura phase for the case of migraine with aura. When vomiting is present, rectal forms of analgesics and use of antiemetics might be suggested. It is noted that paracetamol (1 g) on its own has lower efficacy and it should not be considered as first-line treatment alone. Opioids are thought to be ineffective and potentially addictive; thus, they should be avoided [12].

Triptans are recommended as first-line treatment for patients with moderate-severe migraine attacks, or where analgesics failed. Triptans are more effective when administered while headache is mild, but their use during aura is controversial for safety reasons. Combination therapy using triptans and NSAIDs should also be considered when triptans alone are not efficient to control migraine attacks. Subcutaneously injected sumatriptan (6 mg) should be considered when every other symptomatic treatment has failed, as a rescue medication. Triptans are associated with recurrence of migraine attack within 48 hours in up to 40% of patients that responded and with moderate consistency of efficacy across the attacks. Triptans should be avoided in uncontrolled hypertension, coronary heart disease, cerebrovascular disease or peripheral vascular disease, multiple risk factors for coronary or cerebrovascular disease. Finally, the use of triptans in the elderly should be with great caution due to comorbidities, preferably by headache specialists [12]. There are many strategies from stratified treatment to individual/tailored approach [20]. We suggest that a tailored approach is better as many subgroups of migraineurs exist and many patients exhibit adverse event in one or more therapies [12, 21]. All pharmaceutical symptomatic treatment is summarized in **Table 1**.

Type	Drugs	Action mechanism	Indications	Route of administration	Adverse Events	Recommendation level	Federation Approvals
Disease Specific	Ergots Dihydroergotamine Ergotamine	Activation of 5-HT1B/D receptors located on intracranial blood vessels Affinity for dopamine and noradrenaline receptors	Acute	 IV, IM, SC, Intranasal Oral, Rectal	Nausea Vomiting Paraesthesia Ergotism	Low to Moderate	FDA/EMA approved
	Triptans Sumatriptan Zolmitriptan Naratriptan Rizatriptan Almotriptan Eletriptan Frovatriptan	5-HT1B/1D receptor agonists Induce vasoconstriction Inhibit pain pathways Reduce input to the trigeminal nucleus caudalis	Acute	 Oral, Nasal, Rectal, SC Oral, Nasal Oral Oral Oral Oral Oral	Chest symptoms Nausea Distal Paraesthesia Fatigue	High	FDA/EMA approved
	Ditans Lasmiditan	5-HT1F receptor agonist	Acute	Oral	Dizziness Somnolence Fatigue Nausea	High	FDA approved
	Gepants Ubrogepant Rimegepant	Calcitonin gene-related peptide (CGRP) receptor antagonists	Acute	 Oral Oral	Somnolence Dry mouth Nausea	High	FDA approved
No Disease Specific	NSAIDs ASA Ibuprofen Naproxen Diclofenac Tolfenamic Dexketoprofen Acetaminiphen	Non-selective inhibitors of the cyclooxygenase (COX) enzymes (COX-1/2 isoenzymes)	Acute (Naproxen both as acute and preventive)	Oral, IM, IV, Rectal	Peptic ulceration and bleeds Hemorrhagic cerebrovascular accidents Renal impairment	High	FDA/EMA approved
	Antiemetics Metoclopramide Domperidone	Muscarinic activity D2 receptor antagonist 5-HT4 receptor agonist 5-HT3 receptor antagonist Peripherally selective dopamine D2 and D3 receptor antagonist	Acute	 Oral, IM, IV, Rectal Oral, Rectal	Higher risk of QT prolongation Acute dystonic reactions, Akathisia Mild sedation	Moderate	FDA/EMA approved

Table 1.
Pharmaceutical acute treatment in migraine management.

Type	Drugs	Action mechanism	Indications	Route of administration	Adverse Events	Recommendation level	Federation Approvals
Disease Specific	Anti-CGRP/R mAbs	Monoclonal antibodies	Preventive		Injection site pain/erythema Upper respiratory infection Urinary infection Fatigue Nausea/ Vomiting Joint/back pain Abdominal pain Dysmenorrhea Dry mouth Constipation	High	
	Erenumab	Against CGRP receptor		SC			FDA/EMA approved
	Fremanezumab	Against CGRP ligand		SC			FDA/EMA approved
	Galcanezumab	Against CGRP ligand		SC			FDA/EMA approved
	Eptinezumab	Against CGRP ligand		IV			FDA/EMA approval pending
No Disease Specific	Anticonvulsants	Action on	Preventive				FDA/EMA approved
	Topiramate	(1) voltage-gated sodium channels (2) high-voltage-activated calcium channels (3) GABA-A receptors (4) AMPA/kainate receptors (5) carbonic anhydrase isoenzymes.		Oral	Paresthesia Numbness Fatigue Anorexia/ Weight loss Memory/ Concentration difficulties Renal calculi	High	
	Valproate	Blockade of voltage-gated sodium channels Increases brain levels of gamma-aminobutyric acid (GABA)		Oral IV	Nausea Somnolence Dizziness Weight gain Hair loss Spina bifida	Moderate	
	Beta-blockers	β1/β2 receptor antagonists	Preventive	Oral	Nausea Diarrhea Fatigue Dizziness Bronchospasm Exacerbation of Raynaud's syndrome Bradycardia Hypotension Heart block Sexual/ Erectile dysfunction Alteration of glucose/lipid metabolism		FDA/EMA approved
	Metoprolol					High	
	Propranolol					High	
	Atenolol					Low/ Moderate	
	Nadolol					Low/ Moderate	
	Timolol					Low/ Moderate	
	Bisoprolol					Low/ Moderate	
	Calcium Channel Blockers (CCBs)		Preventive				
	Flunarizine	Selective calcium entry blocker with calmodulin binding properties and histamine H1 blocking activity		Oral	Weight gain Daytime sedation Stomach complaints Dry mouth	High	EMA approved
	Verapamil	Blocks voltage-dependent calcium channels		Oral	Constipation Dizziness Nausea Low blood pressure Headache	Low	FDA/EMA approved
	Angiotensin II Receptor Blockers (ARBs)		Preventive	Oral		High	
	Candesartan	Selectively blocking the binding of angiotensin II to the AT1 receptor			Back pain Dizziness Flu-like symptoms Sore throat Nasal congestion		EMA approved
	Angiotensin Converting Enzyme (ACE) Inhibitors		Preventive	Oral		Low	FDA/EMA approved
	Lisinopril	Inhibits angiotensin-converting enzyme (ACE) antagonist			Headache Dizziness Cough Difficulty swallowing/ breathing Anaphylaxis Hyperkalemia Fatigue Diarrhea		
	Antidepressants		Preventive				
	Venlafaxine	Serotonin-norepinephrine reuptake inhibitor		Oral	Fatigue Constipation Dizziness Insomnia Nausea Headache Dry mouth Sexual/ Erectile dysfunction	Low	FDA/EMA approved
	Amitriptyline	Tricyclic antidepressant		Oral	Sedation Dry mouth Urinary retention Constipation Weight gain Blurred vision Tachycardia	Low	FDA/EMA approved
	OnabotulinumtoxinA	Interruption of signal transmission by the nerve cells to the muscles	Preventive	IM	Neck pain Muscular weakness Eyelid ptosis Injection pain	High	FDA/EMA approved

Table 2.
Pharmaceutical preventive treatment in migraine management.

2.2 Prophylactic management

Preventive treatment of migraine attacks is recommended when attacks are severe or frequent (more than 4 days per month) or there are contraindications, adverse effects, failure, or inadequate response of proper use of acute medication. The aim is to reduce frequency, duration, and severity of attacks and conversely increase the effect of acute treatment. The most important in preventive treatment of migraine is to know when to start the treatment and to manage and monitor the migraine patient, so that the disease does not switch from episodic to chronic, a subform associated with significant morbidity and drug overuse [22] and/or complicate with medication overuse headache (MOH). Today, we have both pharmaceutical and non-pharmaceutical (devices, nutrients, etc.) treatment options in our arsenal.

Prophylactic pharmaceutical treatment include no disease-specific agents, such as beta-adrenergic blockers without partial agonism (atenolol, bisoprolol, metoprolol, and propranolol), calcium channel antagonists (flunarizine), antidepressants (amitriptyline), anticonvulsants (topiramate, sodium valproate), and botulinum toxin for the case of chronic migraine exclusively, and disease-specific pharmaceutical regiments, namely the newly introduced CGRP monoclonal antibodies (erenumab, fremanezumab, and galcanezumab) [12].

Drugs that appear ineffective should be discontinued only after 2–3 months at minimum, in order to achieve and observe efficacy. Failure of one drug does not predict failure of others in a different class. Tapered withdrawal may be considered after 6 months of good control, and should be considered no later than after 1 year [12]. To increase adherence, it is recommended to start with a low dose and slowly increase the dosage to the preferable one.

The anti-CGRP/R monoclonal antibodies have demonstrated good efficacy and excellent tolerability in phase II and III clinical trials with only injection site reactions to be the most common treatment-related adverse events [22].

The available treatments have different efficacy and adverse events/contradictions, and each option must be individualized and tailored in the patient's profile and needs. All pharmaceutical prophylactic treatment is summarized in **Table 2**.

3. Pharmaceutical therapies

As previously stated, the pharmaceutical treatment of migraine is divided into symptomatic/acute (to stop the migraine crisis and alleviate the concomitant symptoms, e.g., nausea, vomiting) and preventive/prophylactic (to reduce the frequency, intensity, and severity of the attacks). Drugs from both categories are further divided into substances that have been designed specifically for migraine and to drugs that are used primarily for the treatment of other diseases (non-specific).

3.1 Symptomatic

3.1.1 Disease-specific

3.1.1.1 Ergots

Ergotamine and dihydroergotamine are the two main drugs of this category, and they exert their action via activating 5-HT1B/D receptors located on intracranial blood vessels. They also have affinity for dopamine and noradrenaline receptors [2]. Evidence shows that dihydroergotamine is more effective than ergotamine.

Nowadays, there are some preparations of ergotamine and dihydroergotamine alone or in combinations (usually with antiemetics or caffeine) [23, 24]. Ergots can also induce medication overuse headache (MOH) with very low doses and their use must be limited to less than 10 days per month. Contraindications are coronary artery disease due to the constriction of the coronal vessels [25], arterial hypertension, and cerebrovascular diseases. Due to their impact on the vascular system, they should not be used in combination with other vasoconstrictor drugs. Other contraindications include Raynaud disease, renal or hepatic failure, pregnancy, and lactation.

3.1.1.2 Dihydroergotamine (DHE)

It is available for oral, intravenous (IV), intramuscular (IM), subcutaneous (SC), and intranasal use, whereas the latter route of administration is less reliable and nasal irritation is a common adverse effect [26]. However, its availability varies across countries significantly. The combination of DHE with antiemetics (where the preparation is available) seems to be effective for the treatment of acute migraine. Intravenous formulation of DHE is very effective and well-tolerated for the treatment of migraine [27]. It is proposed as an acute management of chronic migraine in the primary care to the subgroup of patients who do not respond to NSAID-triptan combinations (1 mg of subcutaneous or intramuscular dihydroergotamine) [26]. Nevertheless, two points must be taken into account: (i) DHE route of administration is mostly parenteral, and self-administration is difficult and takes time for the patient to learn. (ii) It is not clear if the addition of an antiemetic (metoclopramide) in the preparation is responsible for the efficacy of DHE (unknown if there is an additive action) [24]. Doses vary depending on the route of administration, i.e., 1 mg SC, 2 mg intranasal, and 2.5 mg *per os*.

3.1.1.3 Ergotamine

Ergotamine is an ergopeptine and the second migraine drug of the ergot family. The most common combination launched in the market is ergotamine tartare + caffeine. Ergotamine has been in clinical practice over 70 years, but there is no common ground for the use of this agent. There are many trials in the literature, which attempts to validate the efficacy of ergotamine. It is recommended for the treatment of acute headache, only in patients with prolonged attacks (>48 hours) or in whom headache recurrence is a substantial issue [28]. This recommendation is in accordance with the European Federation of Neurological Societies' (EFNS) guidelines [20]. EFNS also stated that status migrainosus can be treated by dihydroergotamine (low level of evidence). In many clinical trials [29–32], ergot derivatives showed lower efficacy than triptans and more adverse events (AE). Therefore, these substances should be dealt with caution [2]. Major AEs are nausea, vomiting, and should be avoided in patients who report these common associated symptoms of migraine, or later than >2 hours after the onset of migraine when the gastric stasis has already occurred. Other AEs are paraesthesia, and ergotism (due to long-term use or ergot derivatives).

3.1.1.4 Triptans

Triptans are 5-HT1B/1D receptor agonists and very effective for the acute management of migraine. They are specific to treat migraine as they act at the pathophysiology of migraine, inducing vasoconstriction, inhibiting pain pathways, and reducing the input to the trigeminal nucleus caudalis. There are many available triptans, i.e., sumatriptan, naratriptan, zolmitriptan, rizatriptan, almotriptan, eletriptan, and frovatriptan. With the exception of sumatriptan (oral, subcutaneous, and intranasal) and zolmitriptan (oral and intranasal), the other triptans are for oral use only. Generally, triptans are recommended for moderate to severe attacks and there is good evidence (level A) that combining a NSAID with a triptan will prevent from migraine recurrence [2, 12, 20, 21]. The choice of triptan is and should be individualized. Triptans have different pharmacokinetic and pharmacodynamic profile. Subcutaneous sumatriptan (6 mg) is more effective than oral sumatriptan and is preferred when associated symptoms, such as nausea and vomiting, occur. Intranasal spray has fewer side effects than intramuscular sumatriptan (discomfort, nasal irritation, and unpleasant taste). Comparative studies show that eletriptan has the highest efficacy with short-term and sustained effect. The above conclusion is consistent in many studies. Rizatriptan and zolmitriptan are thought to come in second and third place, respectively, in terms of efficacy, although further analysis shows that sumatriptan, rizatriptan, almotriptan, and zolmitriptan are very similar regarding clinical outcome. Naratriptan and frovatriptan have less but longer efficacy than sumatriptan and are relatively safer than other triptans. Naratriptan, frovatriptan, and almotriptan are also preferred for symptomatic treatment in patients that migraine attack recurs after successful treatment (pain free and most bothersome symptom free in 2 hours posttreatment) [2, 12, 20, 21, 24, 33–36]. Triptans can be given in combination with NSAIDs and the effect is considered to be additive. The most common and well-documented combination is that of sumatriptan with naproxen and is the one indicated for migraine attacks that do not respond to oral high efficacy triptans (e.g., eletriptan 40 or 80 mg, or rizatriptan 10 mg) [21]. Another combination that showed effectiveness in acute treatment is frovatriptan with dexketoprofen. Generally, triptans are safe and effective. Due to the vasoconstrictive action, triptan should be avoided to migraineurs with uncontrolled arterial hypertension, cardiovascular and/or cerebrovascular disease, and peripheral vascular disease. Systematical reviews and cohort studies showed that there is not any correlation between the use of triptans and higher cardiovascular risk, however [37, 38]. Nonetheless, the use of triptans is not recommended in high-risk patients. Finally, as with ergots, the use of triptans should be limited to 10 days per month to avoid medication overuse headache [2, 19–21].

3.1.1.5 Ditans

Ditans are a relatively new and different class of specific acute migraine management. The first and only approved by the Food and Drug Administration (FDA) until now is lasmiditan, a selective 5-HT1F receptor agonist, which shows minimal to zero vasoconstrictor activity in contrast to triptans. It is a suitable candidate for migraineurs where triptans are contraindicated or not well tolerated. Lasmiditan is given orally (starting dose of 50 mg and subsequently increase up to 200 mg if there is no benefit). Because lasmiditan penetrates the blood-brain barrier; it presents common AEs from the central nervous system (CNS, dizziness, somnolence, fatigue, and nausea) that restricts its use to those who drive or operate heavy machinery [39–42].

3.1.1.6 Gepants

The study of CGRP and its implication to the pathophysiology of migraine has led to discovery of a new class of drugs that are CGRP receptor antagonists. Gepants are suitable for treatment of acute migraine in patients who do not tolerate the triptans or when triptans are contraindicated. The first attempts for the manufacture of these type of drugs led to a dead end, as many of the trials were terminated due to hepatotoxicity. Now, we have two gepants that received FDA approval, ubrogepant (2019) and rimegepant (2020) for the treatment of acute migraine in adult patients. However, more clinical trials and real-world evidence are needed to prove their efficacy and tolerability [43].

3.1.2 No disease-specific

3.1.2.1 Nonsteroidal anti-inflammatory drugs

The most well-studied drugs of this category include acetylsalicylic acid (ASA) (aspirin 900–1000 mg), ibuprofen (200–800 mg), naproxen (275–825 mg), diclofenac (50–100 mg), tolfenamic acid (200 mg), and dexketoprofen (50 mg) [44–51]. The difference in dosage depends on the available formulation for each country and the proposed guidelines of each Headache Society [2, 12, 20, 21, 24]. The use of NSAID should be as soon as possible to achieve maximal effect and to preempt the gastric stasis. If the migraineur does experiences nausea or vomiting, parenteral formulations (suppository, intramuscular, and intravenous) of the above drugs should be given with combination of a prokinetic (see below Prokinetics) [12]. For moderate to severe attacks, combinations of NSAID with triptans are recommended. All NSAIDs have more or less (depends on the COX-2 selectivity) the same adverse events including GI bleeds, peptic ulceration, hemorrhagic cerebrovascular accidents, and renal impairment. They should not be given in patients with uncontrolled hypertension or history of peptic ulcer. In case of peptic ulcer, they can be prescribed for a small period of time together with protein pump inhibitors (PPIs).

3.1.2.2 Acetaminophen

Acetaminophen (paracetamol 1000 mg) is a NSAID with different mechanism of action. It is effective in some patients although it has weaker recommendation than NSAIDs for the management of acute headache [12]. On the other hand, the combination of paracetamol with ASA and caffeine is more effective than single drugs and is recommended for the treatment of mild to moderate severity attacks [20, 21, 52–54].

3.1.2.3 Antiemetics/Prokinetics

Many antiemetics (metoclopramide, domperidone, chlorpromazine, prochlorperazine, droperidol, ondansetron, and granisetron) have been studied for the treatment of acute migraine, both as monotherapy as well as adjuvants. The main action as prokinetics is via their dopamine receptor antagonism. Many of them show anti-migrainous action. With the exception of metoclopramide and domperidone, the other antiemetics have a higher risk of QT prolongation and higher rates of acute dystonic reactions, akathisia (extrapyramidal action) and mild sedation, and besides their efficacy (even some of them over triptans) [55–59], they are not recommended for the treatment of migraine. On the other hand, metoclopramide is a mild analgesic when given orally and more efficient when given intravenously. Despite monotherapy with antiemetics is not recommended, adjuvant therapy [45], especially when associative symptoms like nausea or vomiting are present, or latter in the course of migraine (gastric stasis has already occurred), is strongly suggested. The usual dose is for domperidone 10 mg (supportive evidence of efficacy is for 20 mg) up to three times per day or 30 mg (by suppository up to twice per day) and for metoclopramide 10 mg (up to three times per day). Metoclopramide

20 mg is recommended for adults and adolescents, whereas domperidone 10 mg for children due to the possible side effects (dyskinesia, akathisia) [12, 20].

3.1.2.4 Other drugs

Other drugs with low level of evidence that are found to be effective in the acute treatment of migraine attacks are intravenous valproate (dose up to 800 mg) [60–62], adjunctive therapy with parenteral dexamethasone (intramuscular or intravenous) for treatment of acute migraine and status migrainosus [20, 21, 63, 64], and a combination of paracetamol with intravenous tramadol [65].

3.2 Prophylactic medications

3.2.1 Disease-specific

3.2.1.1 Anti-calcitonin-gene-related peptide/receptor monoclonal antibodies (anti-CGRP/R mAbs)

All four anti-CGRP/R mAbs share several pharmacokinetic advantages over small anti-CGRP/R molecules (e.g., greater target specificity and prolonged half-life, making them suitable for monthly administration to prevent migraine). Three of these macromolecules target the CGRP ligand (fremanezumab, galcanezumab, and eptinezumab), while a fourth (erenumab) targets the CGRP receptor [66–68]. They require parenteral administration and have a preferential peripheral site of action, since only 0.1–0.5% of the mAb cross the blood–brain barrier due to their large size (molecular weight around 150 kDa) [66, 69–72]. All four mAbs have shown particular effectiveness for the prevention of both episodic and chronic migraine [71, 72]. Besides the initial skepticism regarding their safety and their potential cardiovascular effect (due to preclinical data that came from studying and blocking CGRP,66) and liver toxicity that emerged after the initial failure of gepants, no safety flags occurred during the large program of their development and all four anti-CGRP/R mAbs have shown similar tolerability and safety in Phase II and III trials. The most common AEs, which were reported during clinical trials, are injection site pain, erythema, respiratory infection, nasopharyngitis, sinusitis, influenza, urinary infection, fatigue, nausea, vomiting, joint pain, back pain, headache, abdominal pain, dysmenorrhea, and dry mouth. Real-world evidence revealed constipation as one of the common adverse effects (not in clinical reporting). Anti-CGRP/R mAbs should be avoided in pregnant and nursing women, as well as in patients with psychiatric, pulmonary, and cardiovascular medical history, until more data are available. Regarding their efficacy, there is not much evidence or head-to-head clinical trials to support the superiority of one drug against the other. Due to their mechanism of action, pharmacokinetics, clinical effect, and cost, Headache societies have formulated practical guides on the proper use of anti-CGRP/R mAbs [5, 12, 21].

3.2.1.2 Erenumab

Erenumab is the first drug of the anti-CGRP/R category and the only until now that prevents native CGRP ligand binding to the CGRP receptor. It is an IgG2 antibody and the only fully human anti-CGRP/R mAb. At 70 mg, the estimated elimination half-life of erenumab is 21 days, supporting monthly subcutaneous dosing and, thus, betterment in patient compliance [73–75]. It is recommended for both episodic and chronic migraine, as well as the treatment of MOH [76]. There are two formulations of erenumab (70 and 140 mg) with almost similar efficacy, and there is a suggestion of starting with the lower dose and increase if there is little efficacy [77]. A review of 3 randomized trials and their extensions suggested that erenumab 140 mg monthly might be preferred over the 70 mg monthly dose in patients with EM or CM and prior preventive treatment failures (>2) [77]. It is administered subcutaneously (SC) once per month, thus achieving better adherence among migraine patients compared to oral daily medications.

3.2.1.3 Fremanezumab

Fremanezumab is a fully humanized IgG2 mAb that potently and selectively binds to both α and β isoforms of CGRP [78]. It is effective for the prevention of episodic and chronic migraine. It is administered SC and has one formulation of 225 mg, which can be administered either once per month, or three consecutive doses (total of 675 mg) every 3 months. Both dosage options have shown similar efficacy and adverse events [79].

3.2.1.4 Galcanezumab

Galcanezumab is a humanized IgG4 mAb with a long half-life (~28 days) that binds to both α- and β-CGRP isoforms with approximately equal affinity [80]. Again, several trials have proven its efficacy for the preventive treatment of migraine [81–83]. As the other two aforementioned mAbs, galcanezumab is subcutaneously administered. The suggested starting dose is 240 mg (2 consecutive doses of 120 mg formulation) as a starting dose and then 120 mg subcutaneously every month [84].

3.2.1.5 Eptinezumab

Eptinezumab is the last anti-CGRP/R mAb discovered till now. It is a humanized IgG1 antibody that potently and selectively binds to both α and β forms of human CGRP [85]. The plasma half-life of eptinezumab after an intravenous infusion of 1000 mg is 31 days. There are two clinical trials (PROMISE-1 and PROMISE-2) that support its efficacy in episodic and chronic migraine prevention [86, 87]. Eptinezumab is the only intravenously anti-CGRP/R mAb and the recommended dose is 100 mg over 30 minutes every 3 months. It is not yet approved by the FDA or EMA (under development).

3.2.2 No disease-specific

Several drug classes, originally developed for other diseases (e.g., epilepsy, hypertension), have shown efficacy for the preventive treatment of migraine. Repurposed drugs may lack the disease-specific mechanism of action and have several adverse effects and contraindication, but show comparable efficacy to CGRP mAbs and are less expensive. As with the use of disease-specific treatments, when using nonspecific drugs, our main goal is individualizing our choice, taking into account the clinical characteristics, medical history, and comorbidities of the patient (e.g., sex, weight, anxiety/depression, hypertension, endocrinological disorders, pregnancy, etc.). The main categories are anticonvulsants, antihypertensive and antidepressant drugs, and other agents (e.g., onabotulinumtoxinA, butterbur, coenzyme Q10, NSAIDs, and others).

3.2.2.1 Anticonvulsants

3.2.2.1.1 Topiramate

Topiramate is one of the most studied drugs for the prevention of migraine, with several clinical studies, systematical reviews, and meta-analysis, showing its efficacy for both episodic and (fewer evidence) chronic migraine [26, 88–93]. Usual dosage ranges between 25 and 100 mg daily (in two divided doses) and there is suggestion, with the risk of more adverse events, of increasing the total dose up to 200 mg daily when the effect is suboptimal [2, 12, 20, 21, 26]. Main AEs of topiramate are paresthesia/numbness (results in intolerance), fatigue, anorexia/ weight loss, memory and concentration difficulties, and renal calculi (uncommon but serious adverse effect). It is contraindicated in pregnant women as it increases the risk of facial clefts and lowers birth weight. Due to the weight loss, topiramate is recommended to obese migraine patients [89, 90, 94].

3.2.2.1.2 Valproate

Whereas valproate is indicated for the preventive treatment of episodic migraine, its side effects (nausea, somnolence, dizziness, weight gain, and hair loss) and the contra-indication to women in childbearing age and pregnancy (teratogenic) have limited its use. Usual doses range between 500 and 1800 mg per day and there is limited evidence of intravenous administration of valproate in status migrainosus [2, 12, 20, 21, 95].

3.2.2.2 Other anticonvulsants

Other anticonvulsants, such as gabapentin, have not proven their efficacy for prevention of episodic migraine and therefore are not recommended [96, 97] .

3.2.2.2.1 Antihypertensive

The two major categories of antihypertensive drugs that show migraine preventive effect are beta-blockers and calcium channel blockers. Most of the evidence emerged from studies regarding hypertension reported fewer headaches in the intervention group vs. the placebo group [98].

3.2.2.3 Beta-blockers

Beta-blockers that are available in almost every country and are recommended from almost all Headache Societies for the preventive treatment of episodic migraine are metoprolol (50–200 mg daily) and propranolol (40–240 mg daily). Other beta-blockers with fewer studies are atenolol (25–100 mg daily), nadolol (20–240 mg daily), timolol (10–30 mg daily), and bisoprolol (5–10 mg daily). Beta-blockers are recommended in hypertensive patients who are under 60 years old or nonsmokers [94, 99, 100]. Due to their mechanism of action and their dosage that is proven to be efficacious for migraine prevention, are not well tolerated and are contraindicated in patients with bradycardia, low blood pressure, cardiac conduction blocks, asthma, depression, and Raynaud phenomenon [2, 12, 20, 21, 101].

3.2.2.4 Calcium channel blockers

The only drug of this category with good level of evidence is flunarizine, a non-specific calcium channel blocker, with calmodulin binding properties and histamine

H1 blocking activity. Recommended dose ranges between 5 and 10 mg daily and is prescribed to hypertensive patients older than 60 or smokers, as well as to patients with Raynaud syndrome. The most common AEs are weight gain, daytime sedation, stomach complaints, and dry mouth, and while there are reports of depression and extrapyramidal symptoms, there is no confirmation [102]. Verapamil is another calcium channel blocker with migraine preventive properties, but it has conflicting supporting data and many Headache Societies do not accept its use for episodic migraine [2, 12, 20, 21, 103].

3.2.3 Angiotensin receptor blockers (ARBs)/angiotensin converting enzyme (ACE) inhibitors

There is also data supporting the use of ACE inhibitors and ARBs as preventive migraine treatments. Candesartan, a specific ARB, has shown positive results in small-scale crossover studies and is used for migraine prophylaxis (16–32 mg) [104, 105]. The most common AEs include back pain, dizziness, flu-like symptoms, sore throat, and nasal congestion. Similarly, a small-scale double-blind cross-over study, found lisinopril (ACE inhibitor) to be effective in episodic migraine [106]. The above data are not universally approved [2, 12, 20, 21].

3.2.3.1 Antidepressants

Antidepressants are recommended as a second-line drugs with level B documentation [20]. The two drugs of this category are amitriptyline and venlafaxine. Among the two amitriptyline, a tricyclic antidepressant has been studied the most [103]. The usual dose ranges between 10 and 150 mg. Its sedative properties have limited its use and it is suggested only at bedtime and especially to those who suffer from insomnia. It also has a place as a second choice drug for chronic migraine [26]. Except sedation, amitriptyline's AEs include dry mouth, urinary retention, constipation, weight gain, blurred vision, and tachycardia. Venlafaxine, a serotonin-norepinephrine reuptake inhibitor, has a weaker recommendation as migraine prophylaxis and is preferred to those who suffer from depression and/or anxiety and those who have also tension-type headaches (TTH). The usual dose ranges between 37.5 and 150 mg daily [2, 12, 20, 21, 94].

3.2.4 Other drugs

3.2.4.1 OnabotulinumtoxinA

Whereas many randomized trials did not prove onabotulinumtoxinA's efficacy for treating episodic migraine (EM) and it is not recommended [107–109], data extracted from chronic migraine (CM) trials recommend onabotulinumtoxinA as an effective and well-tolerated treatment. OnabotulinumtoxinA has a good level of documentation (Level A), and there is specific protocol regarding its use (PREEMPT protocol), monitoring of the patients, and evaluating their response. It should be administered according to the PREEMPT injection protocol, i.e., injecting 155 U–195 U to 31–39 sites every 12 weeks. The most common reported AEs are neck pain, muscular weakness, eyelid ptosis, and injection-site pain, and the sub-analysis of the PREEMPT studies found that adverse events decreased over time [26, 110–112]. Its use in CM with MOH is debatable after a recent trial that showed no superiority against acute withdrawal alone [113].

3.3 Non-pharmaceutical therapies

Like the pharmaceutical, the non-pharmaceutical treatments—neuromodulation devices in particular—gain even more ground in the treatment of migraine.

A set of variables arrange this alternative so far, therapeutic approach. First, the pathophysiology of migraine refers to a multidisciplinary spectrum of mechanisms; second, the disease is among the most disabling medical conditions requiring application of all available treatment options; third, the existing medicinal selections (symptomatic or preventative) are related with poor adherence due to safety and poor response rates ; and finally, there is an international movement encouraging non-pharmaceutical interventions in medicine, including the community mitigation strategies. Patients' preferences rate the non-pharmaceutical interventions for migraine highly [3]. All these factors create large space for non-pharmaceutical treatment options in migraine, which can be used alone or as adjunct therapy to pharmacological agents minimizing unnecessary drug exposure. There is good evidence for neuromodulation and biobehavioral therapies, including cognitive behavioral therapy (CBT), biofeedback, and relaxation training. Less evidence suggests physical therapy, sleep management, acupuncture, and dietary modifications.

3.4 Neuromodulation

Neuromodulation approaches for migraine treatment includes invasive and noninvasive ones. Both procedures act by stimulating the nervous system centrally or peripherally, leading to pain relief, either acutely or preventively. They are constantly gaining space in the treatment of migraine and are addressed either to refractory patients or to patients who do not want medical treatment. All neuromodulation devices are summarized in **Table 3**.

3.4.1 Invasive

There are three invasive neurostimulation methods investigated for migraine and available, yet in very limited use because of the high cost of the device, the surgical implementation needed, and the lack of good evidence of efficacy. In addition, their accessibility and reimbursement vary by country significantly. Thus, they are recommended for patients with refractory forms of CM only. The most common AEs include migration of the leads, infection, and paraesthesias [7].

3.4.2 Invasive occipital nerve stimulation (iONS)

Invasive occipital nerve stimulation (iONS) has been used to treat refractory CM cases. The exact mechanism of the neuromodulation effect in CNS remains unclear. From three randomized, sham-controlled studies [114–116], only one showed a significant improvement of migraines in the treated group comparing to sham group or the medication treated group [115]. Electrodes must be implanted subcutaneously above the great occipital nerve (GON), which present great anatomical variability among individuals [117]. The leads are implanted bilaterally, while a small generator is implanted subaxillary. The AEs include lead migration, paraesthesias, infections, and battery depletion, but safety data look better than the other invasive procedures [116].

3.4.3 Vagal nerve stimulation (VNS)

Vagal nerve stimulation (VNS) is already applied in patients with refractory epilepsy. The stimulation of vagal afferents decreases the activity of the nociceptive neurons of the spinothalamic and spinoreticular tract, which, in their turn, inhibit the nociceptive transmission in spinal and trigeminal nucleus complex, leading to

Type	Device	Action mechanism	Indications	Route of administration	Adverse Events	Recommendation Level	Federation approvals
Non-Invasive	Supraorbital nerve Stimulation (eTNS)	Regulates peripheral and central pathways of migraine	Acute and Preventive treatment of migraine	Forehead transcutaneously 20 min daily in prevention/60 mins on attack	Allodynia Paresthesia (Minor)	Moderate	FDA approved CE marked
	Transcranial Magnetic Stimulation (TMS)				Lightheadedness Tingling Tinnitus	Moderate	FDA approved
	sTMS	Attenuates the evoked firing rate of thalamocortical projection neurons	Acute Preventive MwA or MwoA	Over Occipital cortex			
	rTMS	Interrupts the brain hyperactivity associated with migraine	Acute and Preventive EM, CM	Over Occipital cortex		Low	-
	Non-invasive Vagus Nerve Stimulation (nVNS)	Antinociceptive on trigeminal nucleus complex nVNS inhibits CSD	Acute	On neck (on route of vagus nerve)	Neck twitching Change in voice Erythema at the site	Moderate	FDA approved CE marked
	Remote electrical Neuromodulation (REN)	Modulate cephalic pain processing, via endogenous analgesic mechanisms	Acute	Applied on the lateral upper arm	Transient sensation of mild warmth Redness/ Numbness of arm/hand		FDA approved
Invasive	Transcranial Direct Current Stimulation (tDCS)	Modulates cortical hyperexcitability	Prevention of EM /CM	Leads applied over visual cortex	Headache Pain Disturbed vision Fatigue	Low	-
	Percutaneous Mastoid Stimulation	May control CSD	Prevention of EM	Leads placed on ear mastoid, over the skin	None	Low	-
	Invasive Occipital Nerve Stimulation (iONS)	Unclear	Prevention of Refractory CM	Implanted subcutaneously implanted leads above GON	Lead migration Paraesthesia Infections Battery depletion	Low	-
	Invasive Vagal nerve stimulation (iVNS)	Inhibits the nociceptive transmission in spinal and trigeminal nucleus complex	Prevention of Refractory CM	Implanted leads over the Vagal nerve	Infection Muscle cramps Local pain Battery depletion	Low	-
	High Cervical Spinal Cord Stimulation		Prevention Refractory CM	Implanted leads	Lead migration Infections	Low	-

Table 3.
Neuromodulation in migraine management.

cephalic pain control. There is data from case series with refractory CM only showing that patients with implanted VNS (iVNS) reached more than 50% reduction in headache frequency and severity [118, 119]. The scarce clinical experience in this field make iVNS not a common treatment option, for the time being, since it is an invasive procedure with adverse effects (infection, muscle cramps, local pain, and battery depletion), though the clinical experience in the field of epilepsy shows to be safe.

3.4.4 High cervical spinal cord stimulation

This invasive procedure trialed in open label studies in patients suffering from CM and showed a significant reduction in headache frequency and intensity in treated patients, but further investigation is required [120, 121].

3.4.5 Noninvasive

Noninvasive neuromodulation devices provide a safe and well-tolerated therapeutical option in symptomatic and prophylactic treatment of migraine alone or in combination with pharmaceutical treatment. Their evidence of efficacy is moderate to good and almost equivalent to that of drug treatments, while their safety profile may outperform them. There are accessibility, reimbursement, and price issues, however.

3.4.6 Supraorbital nerve stimulation

This is a peripheral noninvasive nerve stimulation or an external trigeminal nerve stimulation device which initiates transcutaneously a mild electric current via leads that are placed on the forehead, stimulating supraorbital and supratrochlear nerves. There is evidence of dysregulated central and peripheral pathways in migraine and evidence that external trigeminal nerve stimulation may normalize function of these pathways [122]. Sham-controlled studies showed that 1-hour stimulation with this device reliefs headache pain during a migraine attack significantly [123], while daily 20-minute treatment decreases the monthly migraine days in patients suffering from EM [124]. The device is FDA approved and CE marked as preventive and acute therapy in migraine. Only mild AES are reported and despite some concerns related to the methodology followed in the preventive trial, its efficacy seems comparable to pharmaceutical preventive treatments [122, 125].

3.4.7 Transcranial magnetic stimulation (TMS)

TMS is a well-established and safe procedure already applied in other neurological diseases, modulating the excitability of cortical neurons dependently on the frequency of the stimulus. Thus, only the single-pulse stimulation (sTMS) and the repetitive-pulse stimulation (rTMS) are used to treat migraine.

sTMS is proved to inhibit both mechanical and chemically-induced cortical spreading depression in animals [126]. In addition, sTMS attenuates the evoked firing rate of third-order thalamocortical projection neurons, indicating the probable neuromodulatory effect in migraine [126]. Overall, sTMS interrupts the brain hyperactivity associated with migraine. sTMS devices are portable and patient-controlled and are applied over the occipital cortex in patients with either migraine with aura (MwA) or migraine without aura (MwoA) for acute or preventive treatment. One sham-controlled study showed that sTMS caused higher rates in 2-hour pain relief posttreatment than the sham group in patients with MwA [127]. Open-label studies have shown an efficacy either in acute or preventive treatment in MwA or MwoA [128–131]. The most common AEs recorded in the trials were lightheadedness (3.7%), tingling (3.2%), and tinnitus (3.2%) [131]. The device is FDA approved for acute and preventive treatment of migraine for people aged more than 12 years.

rTMS and especially high frequency rTMS seem to have a positive effect in the prevention of both EM and CM. Treatment with rTMS caused a significant decrease of monthly headache days over sham-treated patients, for both cases of CM [132] and EM [133], but another sham-controlled study did not confirm the results in CM, probably because of a large effect size [134]. Overall, the majority of rTMS studies reported reductions in headache frequency, duration, intensity, abortive medication use, depression, and functional impairment, with no significant adverse events [135]. Further investigation is needed, however.

3.4.8 Noninvasive vagus nerve stimulation (nVNS)

As in iNVS, the nVNS results in an ascending antinociceptive on trigeminal nucleus complex. In addition, nVNS inhibits cortical spreading depression in rats [136]. In migraineurs, the device is applied on the neck, and it produces an electrical stimulus of adjustable intensity, and therefore, stimulates transcutaneously the cervical part of vagus nerve. The evidence of efficacy in symptomatic treatment of migraine is good [8]. One sham-controlled, class 1 study has showed its efficacy in acute treatment of migraine [137], whereas its efficacy in migraine prevention remains debatable [138–140]. It is used in acute treatment of migraine with consisted results similar to the use of NSAIDs or triptans [141]. In a small-size open-label study, nVNS showed promising results as mini-prophylactic treatment of the menstrual migraine [142]. Reported AEs are neck twitching, change in voice, and redness at the site of stimulation. It is generally well tolerated by the patients, however. The portable nVNS device has received FDA approval and is CE marketed for the symptomatic treatment of migraine.

3.4.9 Remote electrical neuromodulation (REN)

Not only cranial nerves but also peripheral somatic nerve stimulation may also modulate cephalic pain processing, via descending endogenous analgesic mechanisms (conditioned pain modulation). There is evidence that the stimulation of upper arm peripheral nerves (median and musculocutaneous) controls cephalic pain [143]. A noninvasive, portable, and wireless device, applied on the lateral upper arm between the bellies of deltoid and triceps muscles, delivers electrical stimuli that alleviate migraine pain [144]. The device has been tested for acute migraine treatment in one randomized, sham-controlled study showing superiority over sham stimulation in achieving pain relief and freedom and relief of most bothering symptoms without significant AEs [145]. Notably, the treatment efficacy is comparable with this of the current use pharmaceutical ones [146]. Its use is contraindicated to patients with other active implantable medical devices and it is FDA approved for the symptomatic treatment of migraine.

3.4.10 Transcranial direct current stimulation (tDCS)

There is some evidence suggesting that tDCS modulates cortical hyperexcitability and therefore it serves as a preventive treatment for CM and EM. The small-size, sham-controlled studies based on both rationales of anodal stimulation (excitatory) and cathodal (inhibitory) on visual cortex mostly have shown positive effect—with limitations—on reduction in monthly migraine days, headache frequency, pain duration, and severity. Contradictions include previous stroke or epilepsy and comorbidity with psychiatric disorders, among others. This procedure is under investigation currently [147–150].

3.4.11 Percutaneous mastoid stimulation

There is evidence suggesting that the stimulation of fastigial nucleus displays neuroprotective, in particular the stimulation of fastigial nucleus elicits long-lasting suppression of periinfarction depolarizing waves and protect rats against cerebral ischemia [151]. Because cortical spreading depression shares characteristics with periinfarction depolarizing waves, it was speculated that this stimulation of this nucleus may be useful in migraine prevention [152]. The new device for this purpose has electrodes that are placed on the bilateral ear mastoid over the skin.

After few open label studies, one sham-controlled showed a significant reduction in migraine days and response rate vs. sham group in patients suffering from EM, without AEs [152]. The device is under development and further studies are needed.

3.5 Nutrient (nutraceuticals)

Nutraceuticals have been defined as, "a food (or part of a food) that provide medical or health benefits, including the prevention and/or treatment of a disease" [153]. There is an increasingly and demanding use of them by sufferers of chronic diseases including migraine [154], for which there is evidence supporting cerebral energy deficiency [155]. Nutraceuticals may cover this metabolic gap in brain, but the equality of data is low to moderate, however.

3.5.1 Riboflavin

Riboflavin (vitamin B2) is an essential component and precursor of riboflavin 5-phosphate, and modulates the electron transport chain, contributing in energy production in mitochondria. There is evidence indicating that oxygen metabolism is impaired in migraineurs' mitochondria resulting in energy insufficiency [155]. Results from placebo-controlled studies showed efficacy in reducing the frequency of headache days in adult migraineurs [156], but not children [157], or when administered as component in compliment [158]. According to available evidence, riboflavin could be suggested as preventive treatment in adults with EM in a daily dose of 400 mg [20, 159, 160].

3.5.2 Coenzyme Q10

Coenzyme Q10 has a similar action with riboflavin. In placebo-controlled studies, CoQ10 reduced the monthly headache days in adults with EM [161] but its efficacy in children and adolescents remains unclear [115]. There is Level C recommendation for its use as prophylactic treatment in EM [20, 160], and strong recommendation from the Canadian Headache Society (CHS) [159] in a dosage of 100 mg TID.

3.5.3 Magnesium

Magnesium deficiency may increase migraine susceptibility. Oral magnesium has been studied in migraine prophylaxis largely [162], as the intravenous $MgSO_4$ for the symptomatic treatment of migraine [163]. Oral magnesium is suggested for migraine prophylaxis with level B or C of evidence [20, 160], in a daily dose of 600 mg. A later meta-analysis downgraded the level of evidence, however [162]. Adverse events with magnesium are soft stool, diarrhea, and flushing. For the symptomatic treatment of migraine, intravenous $MgSO_4$ has failed to show beneficial effect in terms of reduction of pain and rescue medications, while several adverse effects reported questioning the clinical relevance of this symptomatic treatment [163].

3.5.4 Petasites hybridus or Butterbur

Petasites is a herbal extract, with moderate to good evidence of efficacy in migraine prevention [164, 165]. However, there are safety issues related with liver toxicity [166]. Yet, it is recommended as a second-choice treatment for the prevention of migraine [20, 167].

3.5.5 Tanacetum parthenium *(Feverfew)*

Feverfew is a medicinal plant that has been investigated for the migraine prophylaxis with controversial results. A recent review presents some positive findings in comparison to previous ones [168, 169]. Not major AEs are reported (usually mouth ulcers and gastrointestinal complaints). CHS does not recommend the use of Feverfew for migraine prevention; AAN/AHS recommends it as probably effective (level B) and EFNS as possibly effective (level C).

3.5.6 Ginkgolide-B

Ginkgolide-B is an extract from *Ginkgo biloba* tree that has shown efficacy in the prevention of migraine in a small-size, open label study [170], without any other confirmation.

3.5.7 Omega-3 polyunsaturated fatty acids (OPFAs)

The exact mechanism of OPFAs in migraine is unknown. One placebo-controlled study showed no significant difference between active and placebo group in reduction of migraine days [171].

3.6 Dietary interventions

Different types of dietary interventions have been suggested and studied in migraine prevention such as weight loss diet, low fat diets, ketogenic diets, and elimination diets, being the most popular and well-studied ones, and there are reports for several others. Because of the high comorbidity of headache with obesity, weight loss diet is a promising approach linked through inflammatory mediators that are released from adipose tissue. Nevertheless, it does not come out that weight loss or change in dietary intake may attenuate migraine frequency [172].

3.7 Acupuncture

Unrelated to placebo effect, a proportion of patients respond to acupuncture treatment in practice. From recently reviews, acupuncture shows at least not inferior efficacy in the prevention of migraine comparing to conventional prophylactic treatment at a 3-month follow-up vs. placebo, although there is lot of discussion about the high proportion of placebo effect in this procedure (no significant difference between verum acupuncture vs. sham acupuncture groups) [173, 174]. Only minor gastrointestinal AEs are reported. Despite the debatable mechanism of action and the methodological shortcomings of the relative research, the evidence suggests its use in migraine prevention, representing a therapeutic option for those patients who do not prefer medicinal treatments or display nocebo behaviors, which are very prevalent among migraineurs [11]. High recurrence rates after 6-month follow-up have been reported, however [174].

3.8 Physical therapy

The use of physical activity in alleviating the burden of migraine is unclear and data are missing. A cross-sectional study showed that physically active respondents had lower odds of migraine than moderately active respondents [175]. Physical treatment may have an effect, however, several musculoskeletal dysfunctions, in particular neck pain and vestibular symptoms have been reported to coexist with migraine [176, 177]. Thus, physical interventions may improve clinical outcomes when combined with pharmacotherapy. These include manual treatment of trigger points and stretching of the sternocleidomastoid and upper trapezius muscles, among other techniques (e.g., relaxation and aerobic exercise). Although physical therapy is recommended [178], the evidence of efficacy is very limited, and the documentation is rather empirical. A meta-analysis of controlled trials found that physical therapy techniques reduced the duration of migraine attacks but had no effect on pain intensity and attack frequency [179]. Thus, further investigation is needed.

4. Cognitive behavioral therapies

Though it is generally believed that biofeedback, relaxation training, and CBT improve migraine treatment outcomes either alone, or more often, in combination with medications, the evidence is poor. In one randomized trial among young patients (10–17 years old) suffering from chronic migraine, the use of CBT (10 sessions) plus amitriptyline resulted in greater reductions in days with headache and migraine-related disability compared with the use of headache education plus amitriptyline [180]. A recent meta-analysis found that 54% of individuals with migraine reported at least 50% reduction in migraine frequency after psychological therapy, vs. 24% of controls [181]. Because CBT differs substantially from traditional psychotherapy, it focuses on here and now and it is typically time limited; this therapeutic option may help practitioners in migraine management, in pediatric populations in particular [182].

5. Patient centricity and patient education

Migraine is a heterogeneous disease with a spectrum of clinical manifestations varying between individuals. The choice of therapy requires an individual approach, as each patient is unique. Severity and frequency of attacks, disability causing, other symptoms, time to peak, patient preferences, comorbidities, drug interactions, side effects, and prior therapies that failed should be all taken into consideration [2]. Before proposing any therapeutic approach, local availability and accessibility to medications should also be considered. Patient preferences and needs of each individual are essential to achieve treatment adherence and patient-reported satisfaction. Fast-acting drugs are generally preferred from patients with migraine during acute attacks [183]. Effectiveness of drugs seems to be the most important issue regarding prophylactic treatment, followed by time to effect and adverse events [184]. Although patient centricity has been established in the last years, it is not yet a standard practice to include patients at all appropriate levels of decision-making processes that are related to their health and well-being. Patient education is also of great significance to ensure treatment adherence. This could be achieved by thoroughly explaining patients' disorder, purpose, and means of management. Ineffective clinician-patient communication is a major reason for patient treatment nonadherence. Patients thus should be counseled in advance on the potential benefits of the proposed therapy as well as on the treatment-related adverse effects that may appear. In conclusion, clinicians should always individualize their treatment strategy to the specific needs of each migraine sufferer, with multidisciplinary approaches, usually both pharmaceutical and non-pharmaceutical. Patients should be encouraged to take an active role in their own therapy [21]. Due to the heterogeneity of migraine, developers of guidelines should engage patients and patients' organizations to identify and ensure that patient preferences and values are taken into account. Patient engagement should be a major part of migraine care decision-making, avoiding a population level "one-size-fits-all" solution.

Author details

Theodoros Mavridis[1*], Marianthi Breza[1], Christina I. Deligianni[1,2] and Dimos D. Mitsikostas[1]

1 1st Department of Neurology, Eginition Hospital, Medical School, National and Kapodistrian University of Athens, Athens, Greece

2 Neurology Department, Athens Naval Hospital, Athens, Greece

*Address all correspondence to: mavridismdr@gmail.com

References

[1] Terwindt GM. Emerging treatments for headache: Advances in 2019. The Lancet Neurology. 2020;**19**(1):7-8

[2] Mitsikostas DD, Paemeleire K. Pharmacological Management of Headaches. Springer; 2016. pp. 19-28

[3] Mitsikostas DD, Belesioti I, Arvaniti C, Mitropoulou E, Deligianni C, Kasioti E, et al. Patients' preferences for headache acute and preventive treatment. The Journal of Headache and Pain. 2017;**18**(1):102

[4] Tfelt-Hansen P, De Vries P, Saxena PR. Triptans in migraine. Drugs. 2000;**60**(6):1259-1287

[5] Sacco S, Bendtsen L, Ashina M, Reuter U, Terwindt G, Mitsikostas D-D, et al. European headache federation guideline on the use of monoclonal antibodies acting on the calcitonin gene related peptide or its receptor for migraine prevention. The Journal of Headache and Pain. 2019;**20**(1):6

[6] Green MW, Cowan R, Freitag FG. Chronic Headache: A Comprehensive Guide to Evaluation and Management. Springer; 2018. pp. 37-63

[7] Martelletti P, Jensen RH, Antal A, Arcioni R, Brighina F, de Tommaso M, et al. Neuromodulation of chronic headaches: Position statement from the European Headache Federation. The Journal of Headache and Pain. 2013;**14**(1):86

[8] Reuter U, McClure C, Liebler E, Pozo-Rosich P. Non-invasive neuromodulation for migraine and cluster headache: A systematic review of clinical trials. Journal of Neurology, Neurosurgery, and Psychiatry. 2019;**90**(7):796-804

[9] Rehman T, Ahmad S, Fatima Q. Effects of dietary supplementations and herbs on migraine—A systematic review. 2019;**16**(3):20180143

[10] Lee HJ, Lee JH, Cho EY, Kim SM, Yoon S. Efficacy of psychological treatment for headache disorder: A systematic review and meta-analysis. The Journal of Headache and Pain. 2019;**20**(1):17

[11] Mitsikostas DD. Nocebo in headache. Current Opinion in Neurology. 2016;**29**(3):331-336

[12] Steiner TJ, Jensen R, Katsarava Z, Linde M, MacGregor EA, Osipova V, et al. Aids to management of headache disorders in primary care (2nd edition). The Journal of Headache and Pain. 2019;**20**(1):57

[13] Steiner TJ, Lipton RB, Al Jumah M, Al-Khathami A, Allena M, Andrée C, et al. The headache-attributed lost time (HALT) indices: Measures of burden for clinical management and population-based research. The Journal of Headache and Pain. 2018;**19**(1):12

[14] Steiner TJ, Buse DC, Al Jumah M, Westergaard ML, Jensen RH, Reed ML, et al. The headache under-response to treatment (HURT) questionnaire, an outcome measure to guide follow-up in primary care: Development, psychometric evaluation and assessment of utility. The Journal of Headache and Pain. 2018;**19**(1):15

[15] Westergaard ML, Steiner TJ, MacGregor EA, Antonaci F, Tassorelli C, Buse DC, et al. The headache under-response to treatment (HURT) questionnaire: Assessment of utility in headache specialist care. The Journal of Headache and Pain. 2013;**33**(4):245-255

[16] Buse DC, Sollars CM, Steiner TJ, Jensen RH, Al Jumah MA, Lipton RB. Why HURT? A review of clinical

instruments for headache management. Current Pain and Headache Reports. 2012;**16**(3):237-254

[17] Bigal ME, Rapoport AM, Lipton RB, Tepper SJ, Sheftell FD. Assessment of migraine disability using the migraine disability assessment (MIDAS) questionnaire: A comparison of chronic migraine with episodic migraine. Headache. 2003;**43**(4):336-342

[18] Lipton RB, Stewart WF, Sawyer J, Edmeads JG. Clinical utility of an instrument assessing migraine disability: The migraine disability assessment (MIDAS) questionnaire. Headache. 2001;**41**(9):854-861

[19] Headache Classification Committee of the International Headache Society (IHS). The International Classification of Headache Disorders. Vol. 38(1), 3rd ed. 2018. pp. 1-211

[20] Evers S, Áfra J, Frese A, Goadsby PJ, Linde M, May A, et al. EFNS guideline on the drug treatment of migraine—Revised report of an EFNS task force. European Journal of Neurology. 2009;**16**(9):968-981

[21] Kouremenos E, Arvaniti C, Constantinidis TS, Giannouli E, Fakas N, Kalamatas T, et al. Consensus of the Hellenic Headache Society on the diagnosis and treatment of migraine. The Journal of Headache and Pain. 2019;**20**(1):113

[22] Agostoni EC, Barbanti P, Calabresi P, Colombo B, Cortelli P, Frediani F, et al. Current and emerging evidence-based treatment options in chronic migraine: A narrative review. The Journal of Headache and Pain. 2019;**20**(1):92

[23] Capobianco DJ, Cheshire WP, Campbell JK. An overview of the diagnosis and pharmacologie treatment of migraine. Mayo Clinic Proceedings. 1996;**71**(11):1055-1066

[24] Jonathan HS. Acute treatment of migraine in adults. In: Post T, ed. UpToDate. Waltham, MA: UpToDate; 2020 [Accessed: 13 April 2020]

[25] MaassenVanDenBrink A, Reekers M, Bax WA, Ferrari MD, Saxena PR. Coronary side-effect potential of current and prospective antimigraine drugs. Circulation. 1998;**98**(1):25-30

[26] Becker WJ. The diagnosis and management of chronic migraine in primary care. Headache. 2017;**57**(9):1471-1481

[27] Nagy AJ, Gandhi S, Bhola R, Goadsby PJ. Intravenous dihydroergotamine for inpatient management of refractory primary headaches. Neurology. 2011;**77**(20):1827-1832

[28] Tfelt-Hansen P, Saxena PR, Dahlöf C, Pascual J, Láinez M, Henry P, et al. Ergotamine in the acute treatment of migraine: A review and European consensus. Brain. 2000;**123**(1):9-18

[29] Randomized A. Double-blind comparison of sumatriptan and cafergot in the acute treatment of migraine. European Neurology. 1991;**31**(5):314-322

[30] Christie S, Göbel H, Mateos V, Allen C, Vrijens F, Shivaprakash M. Crossover comparison of efficacy and preference for rizatriptan 10 mg versus ergotamine/caffeine in migraine. European Neurology. 2003;**49**(1):20-29

[31] Diener HC, Jansen JP, Reches A, Pascual J, Pitei D, Steiner TJ. Efficacy, tolerability and safety of oral eletriptan and ergotamine plus caffeine (Cafergot®) in the acute treatment of migraine: A multicentre, randomised, double-blind, placebo-controlled comparison. European Neurology. 2002;**47**(2):99-107

[32] Láinez MJA, Galván J, Heras J, Vila C. Crossover, double-blind clinical trial comparing almotriptan and ergotamine plus caffeine for acute migraine therapy. European Journal of Neurology. 2007;**14**(3):269-275

[33] Thorlund K, Mills EJ, Wu P, Ramos E, Chatterjee A, Druyts E, et al. Comparative efficacy of triptans for the abortive treatment of migraine: A multiple treatment comparison meta-analysis. Cephalalgia. 2014;**34**(4):258-267

[34] Dahlöf C. Infrequent or non-response to oral sumatriptan does not predict response to other triptans—Review of four trials. Cephalagia. 2006;**26**(2):98-106

[35] Ferrari MD, Roon KI, Lipton RB, Goadsby PJ. Oral triptans (serotonin 5-$HT_{1B/1D}$ agonists) in acute migraine treatment: A meta-analysis of 53 trials. The Lancet. 2001;**358**(9294):1668-1675

[36] Johnston MM, Rapoport AM. Triptans for the management of migraine. Drugs. 2010;**70**(12):1505-1518

[37] Roberto G, Raschi E, Piccinni C, Conti V, Vignatelli L, D'Alessandro R, et al. Adverse cardiovascular events associated with triptans and ergotamines for treatment of migraine: Systematic review of observational studies. Cephalalgia: An International Journal of Headache. 2014;**35**(2):118-131

[38] Hall GC, Brown MM, Mo J, MacRae KD. Triptans in migraine: The risks of stroke, cardiovascular disease, and death in practice. Neurology. 2004;**62**(4):563-568

[39] Goadsby PJ, Wietecha LA, Dennehy EB, Kuca B, Case MG, Aurora SK, et al. Phase 3 randomized, placebo-controlled, double-blind study of lasmiditan for acute treatment of migraine. Brain. 2019;**142**(7):1894-1904

[40] Oswald JC, Schuster NM. Lasmiditan for the treatment of acute migraine: A review and potential role in clinical practice. Journal of Pain Research. 2018;**11**:2221-2227

[41] Kuca B, Silberstein SD, Wietecha L, Berg PH, Dozier G, Lipton RB. Lasmiditan is an effective acute treatment for migraine. A phase 3 randomized study. Neurology. 2018;**91**(24):e2222-e2232

[42] Tepper SJ, Krege JH, Lombard L, Asafu-Adjei JK, Dowsett SA, Raskin J, et al. Characterization of dizziness after lasmiditan usage: Findings from the SAMURAI and SPARTAN acute migraine treatment randomized trials. Headache. 2019;**59**(7):1052-1062

[43] Moreno-Ajona D, Pérez-Rodríguez A, Goadsby PJ. Gepants, calcitonin-gene-related peptide receptor antagonists: What could be their role in migraine treatment? Current Opinion in Neurology. 2020;**33**(3):309-315

[44] Marmura MJ, Silberstein SD, Schwedt TJ. The acute treatment of migraine in adults: The American Headache Society evidence assessment of migraine pharmacotherapies. Headache. 2015;**55**(1):3-20

[45] Kirthi V, Derry S, Moore RA. Aspirin with or without an antiemetic for acute migraine headaches in adults. Cochrane Database of Systematic Reviews. 2013;**4**:Cd008041

[46] Biglione B, Gitin A, Gorelick PB, Hennekens C. Aspirin in the treatment and prevention of migraine headaches: Possible additional clinical options for primary healthcare providers. The American Journal of Medicine. 2020;**133**(4):412-416

[47] Rabbie R, Derry S, Moore RA. Ibuprofen with or without an antiemetic for acute migraine headaches in adults.

Cochrane Database Systematic Reviews. 2013;**4**:Cd008039

[48] Law S, Derry S, Moore RA. Naproxen with or without an antiemetic for acute migraine headaches in adults. Cochrane Database Systematic Reviews. 2013;**10**:Cd009455

[49] Derry S, Rabbie R, Moore RA. Diclofenac with or without an antiemetic for acute migraine headaches in adults. Cochrane Database Systematic Reviews. 2013;**4**:Cd008783

[50] Myllylä VV, Havanka H, Herrala L, Kangasniemi P, Rautakorpi I, Turkka J, et al. Tolfenamic acid rapid release versus sumatriptan in the acute treatment of migraine: Comparable effect in a double-blind, randomized, controlled, parallel-group study. Headache. 1998;**38**(3):201-207

[51] Gungor F, Akyol KC, Kesapli M, Celik A, Karaca A, Bozdemir MN, et al. Intravenous dexketoprofen vs placebo for migraine attack in the emergency department: A randomized, placebo-controlled trial. Cephalalgia: An International Journal of Headache. 2016;**36**(2):179-184

[52] Lipton RB, Stewart WF, Ryan RE Jr, Saper J, Silberstein S, Sheftell F. Efficacy and safety of acetaminophen, aspirin, and caffeine in alleviating migraine headache pain: Three double-blind, randomized, placebo-controlled trials. Archives of Neurology. 1998;**55**(2):210-217

[53] Diener H, Pfaffenrath V, Pageler L, Peil H, Aicher B. The fixed combination of acetylsalicylic acid, paracetamol and caffeine is more effective than single substances and dual combination for the treatment of headache: A multicentre, randomized, double-blind, single-dose, placebo-controlled parallel group study. Cephalalgia: An International Journal of Headache. 2005;**25**(10):776-787

[54] Goldstein J, Silberstein SD, Saper JR, Ryan RE Jr, Lipton RB. Acetaminophen, aspirin, and caffeine in combination versus ibuprofen for acute migraine: Results from a multicenter, double-blind, randomized, parallel-group, single-dose, placebo-controlled study. Headache. 2006;**46**(3):444-453

[55] Orr SL, Aubé M, Becker WJ, Davenport WJ, Dilli E, Dodick D, et al. Canadian Headache Society systematic review and recommendations on the treatment of migraine pain in emergency settings. Cephalalgia: An International Journal of Headache. 2015;**35**(3):271-284

[56] BET 1: Metoclopramide or prochlorperazine for headache in acute migraine? Emergency Medicine Journal. 2013;**30**(7):595-596

[57] Friedman BW, Irizarry E, Solorzano C, Latev A, Rosa K, Zias E, et al. Randomized study of IV prochlorperazine plus diphenhydramine vs IV hydromorphone for migraine. Neurology. 2017;**89**(20):2075-2082

[58] Kostic MA, Gutierrez FJ, Rieg TS, Moore TS, Gendron RT. A prospective, randomized trial of intravenous prochlorperazine versus subcutaneous sumatriptan in acute migraine therapy in the emergency department. Annals of Emergency Medicine. 2010;**56**(1):1-6

[59] Bigal ME, Bordini CA, Speciali JG. Intravenous chlorpromazine in the Emergency Department treatment of migraines: A randomized controlled trial. Journal of Emergency Medicine. 2002;**23**(2):141-148

[60] Mazaheri S, Poorolajal J, Hosseinzadeh A, Fazlian MM. Effect of intravenous sodium valproate vs dexamethasone on acute migraine headache: A double blind randomized clinical trial. PLoS One. 2015;**10**(3):e0120229

[61] Edwards KR, Norton J, Behnke M. Comparison of intravenous valproate versus intramuscular dihydroergotamine and metoclopramide for acute treatment of migraine headache. 2001;**41**(10):976-980

[62] Leniger T, Pageler L, Stude P, Diener HC, Limmroth V. Comparison of intravenous valproate with intravenous lysine-acetylsalicylic acid in acute migraine attacks. Headache. 2005;**45**(1):42-46

[63] Colman I, Friedman BW, Brown MD, Innes GD, Grafstein E, Roberts TE, et al. Parenteral dexamethasone for acute severe migraine headache: Meta-analysis of randomised controlled trials for preventing recurrence. BMJ. 2008;**336**(7657):1359-1361

[64] Singh A, Alter HJ, Zaia B. Does the addition of dexamethasone to standard therapy for acute migraine headache decrease the incidence of recurrent headache for patients treated in the emergency department? A meta-analysis and systematic review of the literature. Annals of Emergency Medicine. 2008;**15**(12):1223-1233

[65] Silberstein SD, Freitag FG, Rozen TD, Kudrow DB, Hewitt DJ, Jordan DM, et al. Tramadol/acetaminophen for the treatment of acute migraine pain: Findings of a randomized, placebo-controlled trial. Headache. 2005;**45**(10):1317-1327

[66] Giamberardino MA, Affaitati G, Costantini R, Cipollone F, Martelletti P. Calcitonin gene-related peptide receptor as a novel target for the management of people with episodic migraine: Current evidence and safety profile of erenumab. Journal of Pain Research. 2017;**10**(0):2751-2760

[67] Wrobel Goldberg S, Silberstein SD. Targeting CGRP: A new era for migraine treatment. CNS Drugs. 2015;**29**(6):443-452

[68] Bigal ME, Walter S, Bronson M, Alibhoy A, Escandon R. Cardiovascular and hemodynamic parameters in women following prolonged CGRP inhibition using LBR-101, a monoclonal antibody against CGRP. Cephalalgia: An International Journal of Headache. 2014;**34**(12):968-976

[69] Edvinsson L. CGRP receptor antagonists and antibodies against CGRP and its receptor in migraine treatment. British Journal of Clinical Pharmacology. 2015;**80**(2):193-199

[70] Edvinsson L. The journey to establish CGRP as a migraine target: A retrospective view. Headache. 2015;**55**(9):1249-1255

[71] Martelletti P. Erenumab is effective in reducing migraine frequency and improving physical functioning. BMJ Evidence-Based Medicine. 2018;24(2):76

[72] Edvinsson L, Haanes KA, Warfvinge K, Krause DN. CGRP as the target of new migraine therapies—Successful translation from bench to clinic. Nature Reviews. Neurology. 2018;**14**(6):338-350

[73] Vu T, Ma P, Chen J, Hoon J, Van Hecken A, Yan L, et al. Characterizing the relationship between AMG 334 concentration and capsaicin-induced increase in dermal blood flow in healthy subjects and migraine patients using pharmacokinetic-pharmacodynamic modeling. Headache. 2015;**55**(0): 175-176

[74] Sun H, Dodick DW, Silberstein S, Goadsby PJ, Reuter U, Ashina M, et al. Safety and efficacy of AMG 334 for prevention of episodic migraine: A randomised, double-blind, placebo-controlled, phase 2 trial. The Lancet Neurology. 2016;**15**(4):382-390

[75] de Hoon J, Van Hecken A, Vandermeulen C, Yan L, Smith B, Chen JS, et al. Phase I, randomized, double-blind, placebo-controlled, single-dose, and multiple-dose studies of erenumab in healthy subjects and patients with migraine. Clinical pharmacology and therapeutics. 2018;**103**(5):815-825

[76] Goadsby PJ, Reuter U, Hallstrom Y, Broessner G, Bonner JH, Zhang F, et al. A controlled trial of erenumab for episodic migraine. The New England Journal of Medicine. 2017;**377**(22):2123-2132

[77] Ornello R, Tiseo C, Frattale I, Perrotta G, Marini C, Pistoia F, et al. The appropriate dosing of erenumab for migraine prevention after multiple preventive treatment failures: A critical appraisal. The Journal of Headache and Pain. 2019;**20**(1):99

[78] Bigal ME, Escandon R, Bronson M, Walter S, Sudworth M, Huggins JP, et al. Safety and tolerability of LBR-101, a humanized monoclonal antibody that blocks the binding of CGRP to its receptor: Results of the Phase 1 program. Cephalalgia: An International Journal of Headache. 2014;**34**(7):483-492

[79] Dodick DW, Silberstein SD, Bigal ME, Yeung PP, Goadsby PJ, Blankenbiller T, et al. Effect of fremanezumab compared with placebo for prevention of episodic migraine: A randomized clinical trial. JAMA. 2018;**319**(19):1999-2008

[80] Vermeersch S, Benschop RJ, Van Hecken A, Monteith D, Wroblewski VJ, Grayzel D, et al. Translational pharmacodynamics of calcitonin gene-related peptide monoclonal antibody LY2951742 in a capsaicin-induced dermal blood flow model. Journal of Pharmacology and Experimental Therapeutics. 2015;**354**(3):350-357

[81] Stauffer VL, Dodick DW, Zhang Q, Carter JN, Ailani J, Conley RR. Evaluation of galcanezumab for the prevention of episodic migraine: The EVOLVE-1 randomized clinical trial. JAMA Neurology. 2018;**75**(9):1080-1088

[82] Skljarevski V, Oakes TM, Zhang Q, Ferguson MB, Martinez J, Camporeale A, et al. Effect of different doses of galcanezumab vs placebo for episodic migraine prevention: A randomized clinical trial. JAMA Neurology. 2018;**75**(2):187-193

[83] Skljarevski V, Matharu M, Millen BA, Ossipov MH, Kim BK, Yang JY. Efficacy and safety of galcanezumab for the prevention of episodic migraine: Results of the EVOLVE-2 Phase 3 randomized controlled clinical trial. Cephalalgia: An International Journal of Headache. 2018;**38**(8):1442-1454

[84] Gklinos P, Mitsikostas DD. Galcanezumab in migraine prevention: A systematic review and meta-analysis of randomized controlled trials. Therapeutic Advances in Neurological Disorders. 2020;**13**:1756286420918088

[85] Dodick DW, Goadsby PJ, Silberstein SD, Lipton RB, Olesen J, Ashina M, et al. Safety and efficacy of ALD403, an antibody to calcitonin gene-related peptide, for the prevention of frequent episodic migraine: A randomised, double-blind, placebo-controlled, exploratory phase 2 trial. The Lancet Neurology. 2014;**13**(11):1100-1107

[86] Ashina M, Saper J, Cady R, Schaeffler BA, Biondi DM, Hirman J, et al. Eptinezumab in episodic migraine: A randomized, double-blind, placebo-controlled study (PROMISE-1). Cephalalgia: An International Journal of Headache. 2020;**40**(3):241-254

[87] Kudrow D, Lipton R, Silberstein S, Cady R, Schaeffler B, Biondi D, et al.

Eptinezumab for prevention of chronic migraine: Results of 2 infusions in the phase 3 PROMISE-2 (prevention of migraine via intravenous eptinezumab safety and efficacy–2) trial (P2.10-006). Neurology. 2019;**92**(15 Supplement) P2.10-006

[88] Shamliyan TA, Choi J-Y, Ramakrishnan R, Miller JB, Wang S-Y, Taylor FR, et al. Preventive pharmacologic treatments for episodic migraine in adults. Journal of General Internal Medicine. 2013;**28**(9):1225-1237

[89] Brandes JL, Saper JR, Diamond M, Couch JR, Lewis DW, Schmitt J, et al. Topiramate for migraine prevention: A randomized controlled trial. JAMA. 2004;**291**(8):965-973

[90] Silberstein SD, Neto W, Schmitt J, Jacobs D, Group ftM-S. Topiramate in migraine prevention: Results of a large controlled trial. Archives of Neurology. 2004;**61**(4):490-495

[91] Diener H-C, Bussone G, Oene JV, Lahaye M, Schwalen S, Goadsby P. Topiramate reduces headache days in chronic migraine: A randomized, double-blind, placebo-controlled study. Cephalalgia: An International Journal of Headache. 2007;**27**(7):814-823

[92] Diener H-C, Agosti R, Allais G, Bergmans P, Bussone G, Davies B, et al. Cessation versus continuation of 6-month migraine preventive therapy with topiramate (PROMPT): A randomised, double-blind, placebo-controlled trial. The Lancet Neurology. 2007;**6**(12):1054-1062

[93] Linde M, Mulleners WM, Chronicle EP, McCrory DC. Topiramate for the prophylaxis of episodic migraine in adults. Cochrane Database of Systematic Reviews. 2013;**6**

[94] Jonathan HS. Preventive treatment of migraine in adults. In: Post T, editor. UpToDate. Waltham, MA: UpToDate; 2020 [Accessed: 13 April 2020]

[95] Linde M, Mulleners WM, Chronicle EP, McCrory DC. Valproate (valproic acid or sodium valproate or a combination of the two) for the prophylaxis of episodic migraine in adults. Cochrane Database of Systematic Reviews. 2013;**6**:CD010611

[96] Linde M, Mulleners WM, Chronicle EP, McCrory DC. Gabapentin or pregabalin for the prophylaxis of episodic migraine in adults. Cochrane Database of Systematic Reviews. 2013;**6**:CD010609

[97] Mulleners WM, McCrory DC, Linde M. Antiepileptics in migraine prophylaxis: An updated Cochrane review. Cephalalgia. 2015;**35**(1):51-62

[98] Law M, Morris JK, Jordan R, Wald N. Headaches and the treatment of blood pressure. Circulation. 2005;**112**(15):2301-2306

[99] Larochelle P, Tobe SW, Lacourcière Y. β-Blockers in hypertension: Studies and meta-analyses over the years. Canadian Journal of Cardiology. 2014;**30**(5):S16-S22

[100] Schumann S-A, Hickner J. When not to use beta-blockers in seniors with hypertension. The Journal of family practice. 2008;**57**(1):18-21

[101] Jackson JL, Kuriyama A, Kuwatsuka Y, Nickoloff S, Storch D, Jackson W, et al. Beta-blockers for the prevention of headache in adults, a systematic review and meta-analysis. PLoS One. 2019;**14**(3):e0212785

[102] Stubberud A, Flaaen NM, McCrory DC, Pedersen SA, Linde M. Flunarizine as prophylaxis for episodic migraine: A systematic review with meta-analysis. Pain. 2019;**160**(4):762-772

[103] Pringsheim T, Davenport WJ, Becker WJ. Prophylaxis of migraine headache. Canadian

Medical Association Journal. 2010;**182**(7):E269-E276

[104] Tronvik E, Stovner LJ, Helde G, Sand T, Bovim G. Prophylactic treatment of migraine with an angiotensin II receptor blocker: A randomized controlled trial. JAMA. 2003;**289**(1):65-69

[105] Stovner LJ, Linde M, Gravdahl GB, Tronvik E, Aamodt AH, Sand T, et al. A comparative study of candesartan versus propranolol for migraine prophylaxis: A randomised, triple-blind, placebo-controlled, double cross-over study. Cephalalgia: An International Journal of Headache. 2014;**34**(7):523-532

[106] Schrader H, Stovner LJ, Helde G, Sand T, Bovim G. Prophylactic treatment of migraine with angiotensin converting enzyme inhibitor (lisinopril): Randomised, placebo controlled, crossover study. British Medical Journal. 2001;**322**(7277):19

[107] Evers S, Vollmer-Haase J, Schwaag S, Rahmann A, Husstedt I-W, Frese A. Botulinum toxin A in the prophylactic treatment of migraine—A randomized, double-blind, placebo-controlled study. Cephalalgia: An International Journal of Headache. 2004;**24**(10):838-843

[108] Elkind AH, O'Carroll P, Blumenfeld A, DeGryse R, Dimitrova R. A series of three sequential, randomized, controlled studies of repeated treatments with botulinum toxin type A for migraine prophylaxis. The Journal of Pain. 2006;**7**(10):688-696

[109] Silberstein S, Mathew N, Saper J, Jenkins S, Group ftBMCR. Botulinum toxin type A as a migraine preventive treatment. Headache. 2000;**40**(6):445-450

[110] Aurora SK, Dodick DW, Diener H-C, DeGryse RE, Turkel CC, Lipton RB, et al. OnabotulinumtoxinA for chronic migraine: Efficacy, safety, and tolerability in patients who received all five treatment cycles in the PREEMPT clinical program. Acta Neurologica Scandinavica. 2014;**129**(1):61-70

[111] Diener H-C, Dodick DW, Turkel CC, Demos G, DeGryse RE, Earl NL, et al. Pooled analysis of the safety and tolerability of onabotulinumtoxinA in the treatment of chronic migraine. European Journal of Neurology. 2014;**21**(6):851-859

[112] Bendtsen L, Sacco S, Ashina M, Mitsikostas D, Ahmed F, Pozo-Rosich P, et al. Guideline on the use of onabotulinumtoxinA in chronic migraine: A consensus statement from the European Headache Federation. The Journal of Headache and Pain. 2018;**19**(1):91

[113] Pijpers JA, Kies DA, Louter MA, van Zwet EW, Ferrari MD, Terwindt GM. Acute withdrawal and botulinum toxin A in chronic migraine with medication overuse: A double-blind randomized controlled trial. Brain. 2019;**142**(5):1203-1214

[114] Lipton R, Goadsby P, Cady R, Aurora S, Grosberg B, Freitag F, et al. PRISM study: occipital nerve stimulation for treatment-refractory migraine: PO47. Cephalalgia: An International Journal of Headache. 2009;**29**:30

[115] Saper JR, Dodick DW, Silberstein SD, McCarville S, Sun M, Goadsby PJ. Occipital nerve stimulation for the treatment of intractable chronic migraine headache: ONSTIM feasibility study. Cephalalgia: An International Journal of Headache. 2011;**31**(3):271-285

[116] Silberstein SD, Dodick DW, Saper J, Huh B, Slavin KV, Sharan A, et al. Safety and efficacy of peripheral nerve stimulation of the occipital nerves for the management of chronic

migraine: Results from a randomized, multicenter, double-blinded, controlled study. Cephalalgia: An International Journal of Headache. 2012;**32**(16):1165-1179

[117] Natsis K, Baraliakos X, Appell HJ, Tsikaras P, Gigis I, Koebke J. The course of the greater occipital nerve in the suboccipital region: A proposal for setting landmarks for local anesthesia in patients with occipital neuralgia. Clinical Anatomy. 2006;**19**(4):332-336

[118] Hord ED, Evans MS, Mueed S, Adamolekun B, Naritoku DK. The effect of vagus nerve stimulation on migraines. The Journal of Pain. 2003;**4**(9):530-534

[119] Lenaerts M, Oommen K, Couch J, Skaggs V. Can vagus nerve stimulation help migraine? Cephalalgia: An International Journal of Headache. 2008;**28**(4):392-395

[120] De Agostino R, Federspiel B, Cesnulis E, Sandor PS. High-cervical spinal cord stimulation for medically intractable chronic migraine. Neuromodulation. 2015;**18**(4):289-296

[121] Arcioni R, Palmisani S, Mercieri M, Vano V, Tigano S, Smith T, et al. Cervical 10 kHz spinal cord stimulation in the management of chronic, medically refractory migraine: A prospective, open-label, exploratory study. European Journal of Pain. 2016;**20**(1):70-78

[122] Lauritsen CG, Silberstein SD. Rationale for electrical parameter determination in external trigeminal nerve stimulation (eTNS) for migraine: A narrative review. Cephalalgia: An International Journal of Headache. 2019;**39**(6):750-760

[123] Chou DE, Shnayderman Yugrakh M, Winegarner D, Rowe V, Kuruvilla D, Schoenen J. Acute migraine therapy with external trigeminal neurostimulation (ACME): A randomized controlled trial. Cephalalgia: An International Journal of Headache. 2019;**39**(1):3-14

[124] Schoenen J, Vandersmissen B, Jeangette S, Herroelen L, Vandenheede M, Gérard P, et al. Migraine prevention with a supraorbital transcutaneous stimulator. A randomized controlled trial. Neurology. 2013;**80**(8):697-704

[125] Mitsikostas DD, Rapoport AM. New players in the preventive treatment of migraine. BMC Medicine. 2015;**13**(1):279

[126] Andreou AP, Holland PR, Akerman S, Summ O, Fredrick J, Goadsby PJ. Transcranial magnetic stimulation and potential cortical and trigeminothalamic mechanisms in migraine. Brain. 2016;**139**(7):2002-2014

[127] Lipton RB, Dodick DW, Silberstein SD, Saper JR, Aurora SK, Pearlman SH, et al. Single-pulse transcranial magnetic stimulation for acute treatment of migraine with aura: A randomised, double-blind, parallel-group, sham-controlled trial. The Lancet Neurology. 2010;**9**(4):373-380

[128] Clarke BM, Upton ARM, Kamath MV, Al-Harbi T, Castellanos CM. Transcranial magnetic stimulation for migraine: clinical effects. The Journal of Headache and Pain. 2006;**7**(5):341-346

[129] Bhola R, Kinsella E, Giffin N, Lipscombe S, Ahmed F, Weatherall M, et al. Single-pulse transcranial magnetic stimulation (sTMS) for the acute treatment of migraine: Evaluation of outcome data for the UK post market pilot program. The Journal of Headache and Pain. 2015;**16**(1):51

[130] Irwin SL, Qubty W, Allen IE, Patniyot I, Goadsby PJ, Gelfand AA. Transcranial magnetic stimulation for migraine prevention in adolescents: A pilot open-label study. Headache. 2018;**58**(5):724-731

[131] Starling AJ, Tepper SJ, Marmura MJ, Shamim EA, Robbins MS, Hindiyeh N, et al. A multicenter, prospective, single arm, open label, observational study of sTMS for migraine prevention (ESPOUSE Study). Cephalalgia: An International Journal of Headache. 2018;**38**(6):1038-1048

[132] Brighina F, Piazza A, Vitello G, Aloisio A, Palermo A, Daniele O, et al. rTMS of the prefrontal cortex in the treatment of chronic migraine: A pilot study. Journal of the Neurological Sciences. 2004;**227**(1):67-71

[133] Misra UK, Kalita J, Bhoi SK. High-rate repetitive transcranial magnetic stimulation in migraine prophylaxis: A randomized, placebo-controlled study. Journal of Neurology. 2013;**260**(11):2793-2801

[134] Conforto AB, Amaro E, Gonçalves AL, Mercante JP, Guendler VZ, Ferreira JR, et al. Randomized, proof-of-principle clinical trial of active transcranial magnetic stimulation in chronic migraine. Cephalalgia: An International Journal of Headache. 2014;**34**(6):464-472

[135] Stilling JM, Monchi O, Amoozegar F, Debert CT. Transcranial magnetic and direct current stimulation (TMS/tDCS) for the treatment of headache: A systematic review. Headache. 2019;**59**(3):339-357

[136] Morais A, Liu TT, Qin T, Sadhegian H, Ay I, Yagmur D, et al. Vagus nerve stimulation inhibits cortical spreading depression exclusively through central mechanisms. Pain. 2020;161(7):1661-1669

[137] Tassorelli C, Grazzi L, de Tommaso M, Pierangeli G, Martelletti P, Rainero I, et al. Noninvasive vagus nerve stimulation as acute therapy for migraine. The randomized PRESTO study. Neurology. 2018;**91**(4):e364-e373

[138] Silberstein SD, Calhoun AH, Lipton RB, Grosberg BM, Cady RK, Dorlas S, et al. Chronic migraine headache prevention with noninvasive vagus nerve stimulation. The EVENT study. 2016;**87**(5):529-538

[139] Diener H-C, Charles A, Goadsby PJ, Holle D. New therapeutic approaches for the prevention and treatment of migraine. The Lancet Neurology. 2015;**14**(10):1010-1022

[140] Diener H-C, Goadsby PJ, Ashina M, Al-Karagholi MA-M, Sinclair A, Mitsikostas D, et al. Non-invasive vagus nerve stimulation (nVNS) for the preventive treatment of episodic migraine: The multicentre, double-blind, randomised, sham-controlled PREMIUM trial. 2019;**39**(12):1475-1487

[141] Martelletti P, Barbanti P, Grazzi L, Pierangeli G, Rainero I, Geppetti P, et al. Consistent effects of non-invasive vagus nerve stimulation (nVNS) for the acute treatment of migraine: Additional findings from the randomized, sham-controlled, double-blind PRESTO trial. The Journal of Headache and Pain. 2018;**19**(1):101

[142] Grazzi L, Egeo G, Calhoun AH, McClure CK, Liebler E, Barbanti P. Non-invasive vagus nerve stimulation (nVNS) as mini-prophylaxis for menstrual/menstrually related migraine: An open-label study. The Journal of Headache and Pain. 2016;**17**(1):91

[143] Nir RR, Yarnitsky D. Conditioned pain modulation. Current Opinion in Supportive and Palliative Care. 2015;**9**(2):131-137

[144] Yarnitsky D, Volokh L, Ironi A, Weller B, Shor M, Shifrin A, et al. Nonpainful remote electrical stimulation alleviates episodic migraine pain. Neurology. 2017;**88**(13):1250-1255

[145] Yarnitsky D, Dodick DW, Grosberg BM, Burstein R, Ironi A, Harris D, et al. Remote electrical neuromodulation (REN) relieves acute migraine: A randomized, double-blind, placebo-controlled, multicenter trial. Headache. 2019;**59**(8):1240-1252

[146] Rapoport AM, Bonner JH, Lin T, Harris D, Gruper Y, Ironi A, et al. Remote electrical neuromodulation (REN) in the acute treatment of migraine: A comparison with usual care and acute migraine medications. The Journal of Headache and Pain. 2019;**20**(1):83

[147] DaSilva AF, Mendonca ME, Zaghi S, Lopes M, DosSantos MF, Spierings EL, et al. tDCS-induced analgesia and electrical fields in pain-related neural networks in chronic migraine. Headache. 2012;**52**(8):1283-1295

[148] Antal A, Kriener N, Lang N, Boros K, Paulus W. Cathodal transcranial direct current stimulation of the visual cortex in the prophylactic treatment of migraine. Cephalalgia. 2011;**31**(7):820-828

[149] Przeklasa-Muszyńska A, Kocot-Kępska M, Dobrogowski J, Wiatr M, Mika J. Transcranial direct current stimulation (tDCS) and its influence on analgesics effectiveness in patients suffering from migraine headache. Pharmacological Reports. 2017;**69**(4):714-721

[150] Auvichayapat P, Janyacharoen T, Rotenberg A, Tiamkao S, Krisanaprakornkit T, Sinawat S, et al. Migraine prophylaxis by anodal transcranial direct current stimulation, a randomized, placebo-controlled trial. Journal of the Medical Association of Thailand. 2012;**95**(8):1003-1012

[151] Reis DJ, Kobylarz K, Yamamoto S, Golanov EV. Brief electrical stimulation of cerebellar fastigial nucleus conditions long-lasting salvage from focal cerebral ischemia: Conditioned central neurogenic neuroprotection. Brain Research. 1998;**780**(1):161-165

[152] Juan Y, Shu O, Jinhe L, Na Y, Yushuang D, Weiwei D, et al. Migraine prevention with percutaneous mastoid electrical stimulator: A randomized double-blind controlled trial. Cephalalgia. 2017;**37**(13):1248-1256

[153] Brower V. Nutraceuticals: Poised for a healthy slice of the healthcare market? Nature Biotechnology. 1998;**16**(8):728-731

[154] Orr SL. Diet and nutraceutical interventions for headache management: A review of the evidence. Cephalalgia. 2016;**36**(12):1112-1133

[155] Gross EC, Lisicki M, Fischer D, Sándor PS, Schoenen J. The metabolic face of migraine—From pathophysiology to treatment. Nature Reviews. Neurology. 2019;**15**(11):627-643

[156] Schoenen J, Jacquy J, Lenaerts M. Effectiveness of high-dose riboflavin in migraine prophylaxis A randomized controlled trial. Neurology. 1998;**50**(2):466-470

[157] MacLennan SC, Wade FM, Forrest KML, Ratanayake PD, Fagan E, Antony J. High-dose riboflavin for migraine prophylaxis in children: A double-blind, randomized, placebo-controlled trial. Journal of Child Neurology. 2008;**23**(11):1300-1304

[158] Gaul C, Diener H-C, Danesch U, on behalf of the Migravent® Study G.

Improvement of migraine symptoms with a proprietary supplement containing riboflavin, magnesium and Q10: A randomized, placebo-controlled, double-blind, multicenter trial. The Journal of Headache and Pain. 2015;**16**(1):32

[159] Pringsheim T, Davenport W, Mackie G, Worthington I, Aube M, Christie SN, et al. Canadian Headache Society guideline for migraine prophylaxis. Canadian Journal of Neurological Sciences. 2012;**39** (2 Suppl 2):S1-S59

[160] Silberstein SD, Holland S, Freitag F, Dodick DW, Argoff C, Ashman E. Evidence-based guideline update: Pharmacologic treatment for episodic migraine prevention in adults. Report of the Quality Standards Subcommittee of the American Academy of Neurology and the American Headache Society. Neurology. 2012;**78**(17):1337-1345

[161] Sándor PS, Di Clemente L, Coppola G, Saenger U, Fumal A, Magis D, et al. Efficacy of coenzyme Q10 in migraine prophylaxis: A randomized controlled trial. 2005;**64**(4):713-715

[162] Teigen L, Boes CJ. An evidence-based review of oral magnesium supplementation in the preventive treatment of migraine. 2015;**35**(10):912-922

[163] Choi H, Parmar N. The use of intravenous magnesium sulphate for acute migraine: Meta-analysis of randomized controlled trials. European Journal of Emergency Medicine. 2014;**21**(1):2-9

[164] Agosti R, Duke RK, Chrubasik JE, Chrubasik S. Effectiveness of petasites hybridus preparations in the prophylaxis of migraine: A systematic review. Phytomedicine. 2006;**13**(9):743-746

[165] Prieto JMJBTT. Update on the efficacy and safety of Petadolex®, a butterbur extract for migraine prophylaxis. 2014;**4**:1-9

[166] Rajapakse T, Pringsheim T. Nutraceuticals in migraine: A summary of existing guidelines for use. Botanics: Targets and Therapy. 2016;**56**(4):808-816

[167] Holland S, Silberstein SD, Freitag F, Dodick DW, Argoff C, Ashman E. Evidence-based guideline update: NSAIDs and other complementary treatments for episodic migraine prevention in adults: [RETIRED]. Report of the Quality Standards Subcommittee of the American Academy of Neurology and the American Headache Society. 2012;**78**(17):1346-1353

[168] Pittler MH, Ernst E. Feverfew for preventing migraine. Cochrane Database of Systematic Reviews. 2004;**1**:CD002286

[169] Wider B, Pittler MH, Ernst E. Feverfew for preventing migraine. Cochrane Database of Systematic Reviews. 2015;**4**:CD002286

[170] Usai S, Grazzi L, Bussone G. Gingkolide B as migraine preventive treatment in young age: Results at 1-year follow-up. Neurological Sciences. 2011;**32**(1):197-199

[171] Pradalier A, Bakouche P, Baudesson G, Delage A, Cornaille-Lafage G, Launay J, et al. Failure of omega-3 polyunsaturated fatty acids in prevention of migraine: A double-blind study versus placebo. Neurological Sciences : Official Journal of the Italian Neurological Society and of the Italian Society of Clinical Neurophysiology. 2001;**21**(8):818-822

[172] Evans WE, Raynor HA, Howie W, Lipton RB, Thomas GJ, Wing RR,

et al. Associations between lifestyle intervention-related changes in dietary targets and migraine headaches among women in the Women's Health and Migraine (WHAM) randomized controlled trial. Cephalalgia. 2020;**6**(2):119-125

[173] Trinh KV, Diep D, Chen KJQ. Systematic review of episodic migraine prophylaxis: Efficacy of conventional treatments used in comparisons with acupuncture. Medical Acupuncture. 2019;**31**(2):85-97

[174] Linde K, Allais G, Brinkhaus B, Fei Y, Mehring M, Vertosick EA, et al. Acupuncture for the prevention of episodic migraine. Cochrane Database of Systematic Reviews. 2016;**6**:CD001218

[175] Hammond NG, Colman I. The role of positive health behaviors in the relationship between early life stress and migraine. Headache. 2020;60(6):1111-1123

[176] Lampl C, Rudolph M, Deligianni CI, Mitsikostas DD. Neck pain in episodic migraine: Premonitory symptom or part of the attack? The Journal of Headache and Pain. 2015;**16**(1):80

[177] Ashina S, Bendtsen L, Lyngberg AC, Lipton RB, Hajiyeva N, Jensen R. Prevalence of neck pain in migraine and tension-type headache: A population study. The Journal of Headache and Pain. 2015;**35**(3):211-219

[178] Kropp P, Meyer B, Meyer W, Dresler T. An update on behavioral treatments in migraine—Current knowledge and future options. Expert Review of Neurotherapeutics. 2017;**17**(11):1059-1068

[179] Luedtke K, Allers A, Schulte LH, May A. Efficacy of interventions used by physiotherapists for patients with headache and migraine—Systematic review and meta-analysis. 2016;**36**(5):474-492

[180] Powers SW, Kashikar-Zuck SM, Allen JR, LeCates SL, Slater SK, Zafar M, et al. Cognitive behavioral therapy plus amitriptyline for chronic migraine in children and adolescents: A randomized clinical trial. JAMA. 2013;**310**(24):2622-2630

[181] Sharpe L, Dudeney J, Williams A, Nicholas M, McPhee I, Baillie A, et al. Psychological therapies for the prevention of migraine in adults. Cochrane Database of Systematic Reviews. 2019;**7**:CD012295

[182] Pérez-Muñoz A, Buse DC, Andrasik F. Behavioral interventions for migraine. Neurologic Clinics. 2019;**37**(4):789-813

[183] Smelt AFH, Louter MA, Kies DA, Blom JW, Terwindt GM, van der Heijden GJMG, et al. What do patients consider to be the most important outcomes for effectiveness studies on migraine treatment? Results of a Delphi study. PLoS One. 2014;**9**(6):e98933

[184] Peres MFP, Silberstein S, Moreira F, Corchs F, Vieira DS, Abraham N, et al. Patients' preference for migraine preventive therapy. PLos One. 2007;**47**(4):540-545

Section 3

The Chronic Face of Migraine - Two Approaches

Chapter 5

Chronic Migraine

Diana Obelieniene, Ruta Pestininkaite and Daiva Rastenyte

Abstract

Chronic migraine as a disease was initially recognized in patients with a large burden of disability from frequent headaches and a history of prior migraines. Over time, this observation was operationalized into multiple diagnostic criteria with requirements for frequent headache days, typically 15 or more, which, on at least 8 days in a month, have the features of migraine headache. Chronic migraine affects 1–2% of the general population, and about 8% of patients with migraine. Understanding disease mechanisms still remains a challenge. Inflammation and central sensitization play significant role in the evolutive mechanisms of chronic migraine. Treatment of this condition should primarily focus on the prevention. The currently available evidence-based prophylactic treatment options are topiramate, valproic acid, onabotulinumtoxin A and recently developed promising anti-CGRP monoclonal antibodies. Chronic migraine research is a dynamic and rapidly advancing area. New developments in this field have the potential to improve the diagnosis, to provide more personalized treatments and to reduce burden of disability.

Keywords: chronic migraine, epidemiology, pathophysiology, risk factors, symptoms, diagnosis, treatment, prevention

1. Introduction

Chronic migraine (CM) is a distinct and relatively recently defined type of migraine initially recognized in patients with a large burden of disability from frequent headaches and a history of prior migraine.

The International Headache Society (IHS) defines CM as more than 15 headache days per month over a 3-month period of which more than eight are migrainous [1].

Disability rates and burden of disease among individuals with CM has more-severe impact on socioeconomic functioning and quality of life than does episodic migraine (EM) [2–4]. About 25% patients with CM report a very severe headache-related disability, as defined by the Migraine Disability Assessment Scale (MIDAS) to compare with 3% of patients with EM [2]. The proportion of patients with CM who report reduced household productivity, missed family activities and missed household work is two to three times higher than that of EM patients [4]. The annual per-person costs of CM—consisting of direct costs caused by health care utilization and treatment expenses (~30%) and indirect costs attributable to absenteeism from work and loss of productivity (~70%)—are about fourfold higher than those concerning with EM [5, 6].

Acknowledgment the severe effect of CM on socioeconomic functioning and quality of life, effective treatment of this disorder and preventing progression from episodic to CM—are one of most important problems in management of headache disorders.

IntechOpen

2. History

The current definition of CM as outlined in the International Classification of Headache Disorders, 3rd edition (ICHD-3) [1] is relatively new. This definition has been tested multiple times and has gone through multiple revisions.

Although migraine as a distinct condition of headache with other accompanying symptoms has been known for thousands of years from the early writings of Aretaeus of Cappadocia in 30–90 A.D. [7]. The first formal modern definition of migraine was outlined in 1962 [8]. This first definition did not contain operational rules for migraine diagnosis and in 1988 the IHS published operational diagnostic criteria entitled the International Classification of Headache Disorders (ICHD-1) [9]. Criticism has been raised by experts that the ICHD-1 was not comprehensive enough to introduce diagnostic criteria for chronic headaches [10].

It was recognized in the 1980s that a chronic frequent headache patient population had a history of migraine [11, 12]. The daily and near daily headache patients were classified with multiple diagnoses but likely represented a single pathophysiological entity of migraine transformation with increased frequency. Recognizing this drawback, the Silberstein—Lipton criteria 1994, 1996 were proposed [13, 14]. They stipulated that chronic daily headaches defined as headaches on 15 or more days a month for at least 1 month, there was a subcategory of transformed migraine (TM) [6].

The term chronic migraine the first time in the literature was used by Manzoni et al. [15]. The results of a population study of chronic daily headache patients in Italy showed that 72% had fulfilled an IHS diagnosis of migraine [15]. For the first time CM appeared in the International Classification of Headache Disorders, 2nd edition (ICHD-2), 2004 [16]. There the CM category was defined as a complication of migraine, in patients having migraine without aura on at least 15 days per month, for at least 3 months, before the diagnosis was established. In the comments were stated that chronicity may be regarded as complication of EM and if medication overuse is present this is the most likely cause of chronic symptoms and it was suggested to code probable CM and probable medication- overuse headache (MOH). The requirement of having 15 migraine days per month was likely too stringent [17] and in a field trial of the ICHD-2 criteria [18] only 5.6% could be classified with CM, and only 10% could be classified to probable migraine with probable MOH.

Further, as it was recognized in prior studies, in the process of migraine transformation or chronification, the migraine features of some of the headaches may be lost [11–14].

Recognizing the drawbacks, in an appendix to ICHD-2R the CM definition was specified by requiring only 8 days per month to meet the definition of migraine or be responsive to migraine specific medications. This criterion is still present in the ICHD-3 [1].

ICHD-3 criteria of CM include a mixture of migraine and tension-type-like headaches and do not account for patients with high-frequency migraine attacks in the absence of other types of headaches [19].

Patients with migraine on eight or more days but not 15 days with headache a month are as disabled as patients with ICHD-3 defined CM [19]. Following this data a criticism regarding the existing CM criteria was raised and suggestion to revise the CM criteria was iniciated [19].

3. Epidemiology

The prevalence of CM worlwide ranges is reported to be between 0.9–5% [20], in a general population, and about 8% among patients with migraine [2, 21–24].

However, the true prevalence of CM is difficult to estimate because of heterogeneus data collection instruments.

CM accounts for about one-third of chronic headache (with more than 180 days per year) in general population [23]. This headache disorder is almost three times more common in women than in men with prevalence rate peaks at the ages of 18–29 years with repeating at 40–49 years [2, 22]. Most studies suggest that annually, from about 2.5% of people with EM evolves CM [25, 26], while only a limited portion with CM revert back to EM [25, 27].

The course of CM can change—spontaneous or medically induced remission is possible. About 26% of patients can experience remission within 2 years of the onset of CM [24]. Large-scale epidemiological studies have identified various factors associated with progression from episodic to CM, and also factors that promote migraine remission [27].

Most important nonmodifiable risk factors for migraine chronification are age, female sex and low educational status [2, 7, 14, 23]. Individuals with CM have increased incidence of certain somatic and psychiatric comorbidities—in comparison with people with EM [23, 25]. However, the understanding of complex factors and mechanisms leading to an increased migraine frequency and consequently to the development of CM are only in the beginning and needs further investigations.

4. Pathophysiology

Generally the pathophysiology of migraine is intricate and in spite of substantial progress in recognizing its mechanisms over the past several decades, it still remains not fully elucidated. Even more, so is the pathophysiology of CM. Current evidence defines migraine as a disorder of brain dysfunction with genetic background and environmental triggering [28]. To date there is limited number of scientific studies exploring the chronic form of migraine, therefore the reasons why the disease sometimes takes a turn and attacks become more frequent are not fully clarified yet. The key components proposed in the pathogenesis of migraine chronification include atypical pain processing, central sensitization, cortical hyperexcitability and neurogenic inflammation [29] (**Figure 1**).

Distinct phases of migraine are associated with different anatomical areas and driven by different processes. Prodromal symptoms that can develop prior the onset of migraine pain are believed to be a result of abnormal activity in cortical, diencephalic and/or brainstem areas. Migraine aura, experienced by approximately one third of patients, is most probably caused by cortical spreading depression (CSD)—a phenomenon defined as a slowly propagating depolarization wave followed by a prolonged period of inhibition of cortical activity [28, 30]. Going further, the pivotal process of the headache phase is activation of the trigeminovascular system. As the brain itself has been known to be rather insensate, the intracranial nociceptive impulses are generated in pain-sensitive structures like pial, arachnoid and dural blood vessels, venous sinuses as well as large cerebral arteries, all of which are innervated by nociceptive nerve fibers originating in the trigeminal ganglion. Activation of these structures by various stimuli is responsible for generation of migrainous pain and its associated features [31–33]. Extracranial afferent nociceptive innervation is largely received through the divisions of trigeminal nerve, mainly the ophthalmic, as well as the upper cervical dorsal root ganglia [34]. The intracranial and extracranial neural afferents enter caudal medulla via trigeminal tract and terminate in the spinal trigeminal nucleus caudalis and upper cervical spinal cord (C1-C3)—the trigeminocervical complex (TCC) [35, 36]. Next, the nociceptive information travels further via ascending pathways to the diencephalon

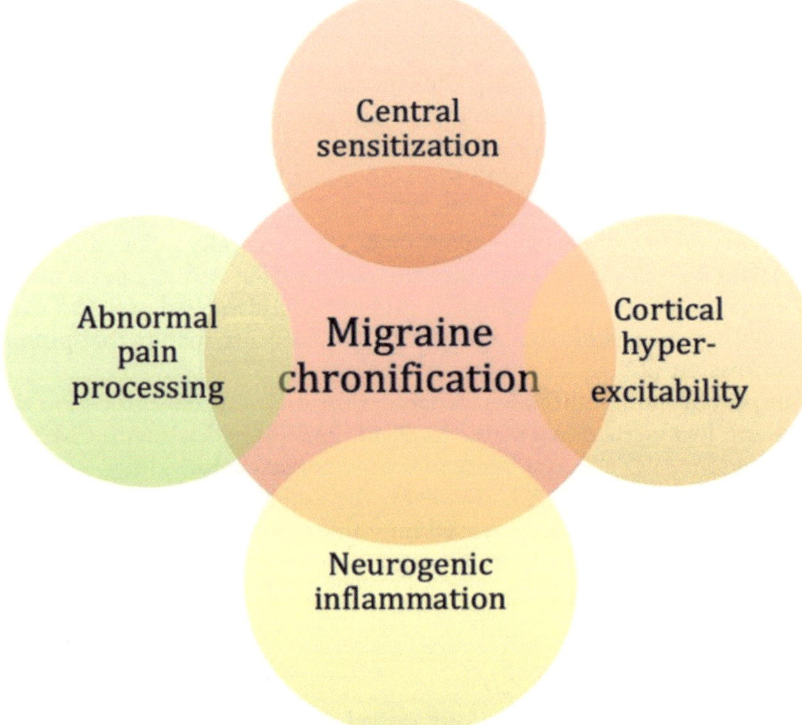

Figure 1.
Components of pathogenesis of migraine chronification. Data from Ref. [29].

and cortical areas, including insula and cingulate cortex. [28] The role of the limbic system is also significant: central pain processing and further relaying of sensory information depend largely on the thalamus [28, 37]; moreover, the amygdala and hippocampus participate in affective and cognitive perception of pain [38, 39]—features contributing to migraine notoriety as a disabling and burden-causing disease with strong emotional implications.

Under normal physiological circumstances activation of the nociceptive system is counterbalanced by pain modulation. It is known that in migraine, descending pain-modulating pathways are dysfunctional and pain inhibition is atypical, therefore susceptibility to migraine attacks is increased [40, 41]. Modulation system originates in the cerebral cortex and is carried out via cortico-trigeminal pathways with participation of brain structures, such as hypothalamus, locus coeruleus, nucleus raphe magnus and rostral ventromedial medulla. A core structure controlling pain and providing endogenous analgaesia is the periaqueductal gray matter (PAG) [42, 43]. Due to repetitive migraine attacks and prolonged exposure to pain, PAG and other structures, comprising the descending pain-modulating network, are excessively activated, which results in oxidative stress and subsequent dysfunction. Thereby adequate pain modulation is not ensured and susceptibility to generation of migraine attacks increases [42–44].

Some authors propose that migraine chronification can be seen as a threshold problem [45]. Pain threshold exists in order to protect from situations where daily non-noxious stimuli could induce pain, therefore it takes a stimulus of certain potency to actually be perceived as painful. Pain threshold is inconstant and shifts depending on cyclic changes that are thought to originate in the limbic system [46]. Those changes allow threshold fluctuations making individuals periodically more susceptible to migraine attacks. During the interictal period threshold is normal, but when it decreases sufficiently, certain events, like stress or changes in hormonal or sleep rhythm, can provoke a migraine attack [47, 48]. Frequent attacks are among the major risk factors of migraine chronification, as they shorten the interictal period thus preventing restoration of the pain threshold to normal level [27, 49]. Consequently the sensory threshold stays below-baseline for most of the time and susceptibility to migraine attacks increases. Likewise, the most common risk factors, as obesity, physical inactivity, psychiatric illnesses and stress, might affect the threshold and make individuals more prone to migraine episodes [45].

Further alteration of pain threshold and increased sensitivity to attack-inducing triggers can be influenced by central sensitization [45]. Cutaneous allodynia, which represents central sensitization, is significantly more prevalent in chronic migraine patients than those with episodic one, suggesting that frequent attacks and higher pain intensity contribute to the development of central sensitization [50, 51]. This also explains why ineffective attack management is a risk factor for chronification: if migraine attacks are not treated completely, it results in a longer and more intense state of pain, leading to pronounced central sensitization, lowered pain threshold and increased susceptibility to migraine transformation [50, 52]. Overuse of acute pain medications is another risk factor for migraine progression, as it has been shown to promote central sensitization and susceptibility to CSD [27, 53].

There has been increasing evidence on altered cortical excitability in migraine [54]. Studies with transcranial magnetic stimulation have demonstrated reduced visual suppression in CM patients compared with EM patients and healthy controls, which proves the presence of cortical hyperexcitability [42]. In addition, assessment of visual evoked potentials shows that interictal excitability of the visual cortex is persistent and matches that of a migraine attack thus creates a "never-ending" migraine [55]. The underlying mechanisms of cortical hyperexcitability have not been uncovered yet, but evidence suggests that it may be induced by dysfunction of the pain modulatory pathways [55].

Another contributor to the pathophysiology of CM is neurogenic inflammation [29, 56]. Upon nociceptive stimulation by chemical, mechanical or electrical stimuli, a number of vasoactive substances are released from the axon terminals, causing vasodilation of the blood vessels and further plasma extravasation, edema and mastocyte degranulation. This so-called "sterile inflammation" results in sensitization and activation of the trigeminal meningeal receptors [28, 56], promoting the induction of migrainous pain [56]. Among the best-studdied vasoactive substances are calcitonine gene-related peptide (CGRP), substance P, neurokinin A, serotonin (5-HT) and pituitary adenylate cyclase-activating peptide (PACAP). CGRP is one of the most significant central pronociceptive agents expressed in the trigeminovascular system and associated with pain processing and migraine symptoms. It takes part in the development of peripheral and central sensitization and enhanced abnormal pain perception [28]. Vasoactive intestinal peptide (VIP) is another important parasympathetic neurotransmitter with a headache-eliciting effect [57, 58]. These pro-inflammatory vasoactive substances have been in the spotlight of research for years with regard to their potential role as biomarkers for chronic migraine. The levels of CGRP and VIP have been measured and compared during the interictal state of episodic and chronic migraine, showing an increase of either in the latter [59]. This provides additional evidence on altered interictal activity of the trigeminovascular system in chronic migraineurs. Moreover, the role of other substances, such as leptin, adipoleptin, TNF-α and glutamate, in the processes related with persistence and progression of migraine, has been demonstrated. This provides reasonable hopes on future implementation of biomarkers for migraine chronification [57, 58, 60].

In terms of anatomic changes in migraine, white matter lesions are considered to be more common in migraineurs than in general population. Moreover, increase in lesions correlates with attack frequency [61]. Recent neuroimaging studies revealed some other neuroanatomical differences correlating with headache frequency that could even be considered indirect markers of migraine chronification: it showed that migraineurs with more frequent attacks had thicker somatosensory cortex, anterior cingulate cortex and inferior temporal gyrus, compared with those with low-frequency attacks [62]. Also correlation with thickness of left middle frontal gyrus and left central sulcus was noted. Moreover, patients with CM had volumetric changes in amygdala, hippocampus, putamen and brainstem areas [63]. These data once again prove the role of these cerebral structures in the pathogenesis of chronic migraine [64].

Genetic influence on the progression from episodic to CM is yet to be established as more large-sample studies are needed [64, 65]. However it looks that chronic migrain has a polygenetic background. Data suggest the role of certain gene groups linked to migraine and pain progression, addiction and medication overuse, hyperexcitability and oxidative stress in migraine chronification [66]. Furthermore, it is becoming clear that epigenetics is also related to migraine as to many other multifactorial diseases. Although to date there are no specific genetic studies in chronic migraine patients, there is some evidence that neuronal activity occuring during CSD may cause epigenetic changes involved in neuronal plasticity, neuroprotection and regulation of basal synaptic activity [67, 68].

5. Risk factors

Not all patients with EM progress into chronic form [69]. The American Migraine Prevalence and Prevention (AMPP) Study [70], the International Burden of Migraine Study (IBMS) [3] and the others have explored at the prevalence of different features in episodic and CM. Some of them have been found to be more prevalent in the chronic form of migraine, suggesting that these features should be seen as risk factors associated with migraine conversion that may serve as prognostic markers enabling prediction of possible migraine progression from episodic to chronic form. Knowing these factors can assist in identifying patients at risk of transformation and take appropriate measures to prevent it (**Table 1**).

The risk factors can be divided into non-modifiable and modifiable. Some of them carry more weight in predisposing CM than the others do. The most significant risk factors are overuse of acute medication [27], ineffective acute treatment [51], obesity [71], depression [72] and stressful life events [27]. The risk factors are listed in **Table 1**.

Studies show that higher prevalence of CM is related to some non-modifiable demographic characteristics, such as female sex [73, 74] and Caucasian race [75]. Regarding age, CM tends to be increasingly more prevalent from 18 to 50 years in both sexes [2]. In terms of the modifiable risk factors, there is evidence for correlation between lower level of education and CM, but data are inconsistent [3, 24, 25, 75]. In addition, some studies propose lower economic status [76], being unmarried [25] and unemployed [3, 25] as risk factors for chronic migraine.

Some modifiable lifestyle features have also been listed as risk factors of CM. First, high caffeine intake is connected with migraine transformation, especially when excessive consumption has started before the onset of chronic daily headache [77]. Second, obesity, especially in women, is more prevalent in chronic than in EM thus it can be considered a risk factor for migraine chronification [71]. In fact, similar relation also exists between increased body weight and other headache disorders like MOH and benign intracranial hypertension [78, 79]. The mechanisms linking obesity and frequent headaches are not known yet, but it may be related to hyperleptinemia [80–82]. Next, sleep disorders, including sleep apnea, snoring, disturbed sleep and oversleeping, have been found to elevate the risk for developing CM [83, 84]. Therefore it is obvious that patient education and counseling on lifestyle is extremely important, as reducing caffeine intake, normalizing body weight and sleeping patterns early enough may help to prevent migraine progression.

Another tendency is that patients with CM report various comorbidities more commonly than those with CM. According to the CaMEO study, patients with the most comorbidities were 5 times more likely to progress to CM than those with the fewest [84, 85]. Psychiatric comorbidities, especially anxiety and severe or moderate depression, are particularly prevalent in CM patients [72, 84, 86] as are some personality traits and disorders, in particular obsessive-compulsive, dependent, avoidant and passive-aggressive [87]. Chronic pain conditions, including fibromyalgia, chronic back and neck pain, are also a strong prognostic factor for migraine progression from episodic to chronic state as they are much more commonly reported by chronic migraineurs [88]. Other comorbidities such as cardiovascular disorders, asthma and allergies [25] are also considered risk factors for migraine progression. Moreover, various major life changes, like divorce, change of employment status or being recently widowed also play a role in migraine conversion, partially by accompaniment of anxiety and depression [27]. Therefore it is critically

Demographic characteristics
Female sex
Caucasian race
Increasing age
Lower level of education
Lower economic status
Being unmarried
Unemployment
Lifestyle factors
High caffeine consumption
Obesity
Sleep disorders
Sleep apnea
Snoring
Sleep deprivation
Excessive sleeping
Headache features
Frequent attacks
Cutaneous allodynia
Treatment-related factors
Acute medication overuse
Insufficient treatment
Comorbidities
Psychiatric disorders
Depression
Anxiety
Bipolar disorder
Personality disorders and traits
Obsessive-compulsive
Avoidant
Dependent
Passive-aggressive
Concomitant chronic pain disorders
Fibromyalgia
Back and neck pain
Painful neuropathy
Cardiovascular disorders
Arterial hypertension
Hypercholesterolemia
Asthma
Stress related with major life changes
Divorce
Change of employment status
Grief

Table 1.
Risk factors for chronic migraine [27, 51, 71, 72].

important to adequately treat these comorbidities in order to prevent migraine chronification, impaired quality of life and development of disability.

In addition to what has been set out before, some headache features have been established as risk factors too. One of the majors is headache frequency [27, 69]. Scher et al. has shown that the risk for chronification increases with the increase of headache frequency in a non-linear fashion. A minimum of three attacks per month is enough to elevate the risk for new-onset chronic headache [27]. This is based on the fact that prolonged exposure to pain induces central sensitization and decreases the attack threshold. Hence this once again emphasizes the importance of rapid and adequate treatment of migraine attacks to prevent pathophysiological alterations leading to migraine chronification.

Another specific clinical feature of migraine attack is cutaneous allodynia, which affects approximately 63% of migraineurs [89]. According to Burstein et al. and Louter et al. it is not only a clinical marker of central sensitization but can also be considered an independent predictor of migraine chronification [50, 52]. From therapeutic point of view, triptans should be administered to terminate a migraine attack within 30 minutes for subjects with cutaneous allodynia in order to minimize exposure to pathological processes leading to migraine chronification [90].

Aditionally some treatment-related factors are proven to play a role in the pathogenesis of CM. The Akershus study [91] among other data has confirmed that acute medication overuse has substantial impact to the processes leading to migraine progression. Acute medication overuse is defined as medication intake on 10–15 days per month [92]. Among the different analgesic groups opioids, barbiturates and combination drugs are associated with the highest dose-dependent risk, while triptans show moderate association with migraine progression and it is more likely in patients with higher baseline attack frequency. Interestingly, some data reports protective effect of NSAIDs against migraine progression, but only in patients with less than 10 attacks per month [79, 92]. The impact of medication overuse in migraine progression is supported by the fact, that attack frequency and disability decreases after discontinuation of acute medication, which also allows more effective preventive treatment [91].

On the other hand, the AMPP study states that ineffective or insufficient treatment can also promote chronification processes [90]. Patients using triptans are more likely to successfully abort the attacks than those using NSAIDs and simple analgesics therefore they are at less risk for chronification [51].

In conclusion it is crucial that effort is made to treat migraine attacks rapidly and adequately as well as to modify other risk factors relevant to the patient so that the pathophysiological mechanisms responsible for migraine progression from episodic into chronic form could be precluded [45, 64].

6. Symptoms and diagnosis

Although the most obvious difference between episodic and CM seems to be the frequency of attacks, clinical migraine features may change too as the disease progresses from less frequent to chronic form. Usually over time the pain becomes more "featureless", thus resembling tension-type headache for most of the time with some more prominent migraine-like attacks interjected [69].

Typical migraine attacks generally manifest as severe, usually unilateral headache of throbbing quality, increasing intensity with physical activity and a combination of associated features: nausea, vomiting, hypersensitivity to visual, auditory, olfactory and cutaneous stimuli. The headache can change sides during or between the attacks [64]. The pain in patients with CM is more commonly bilateral and the associated symptoms are less pronounced than in those with EM [93]. Some patients report prodromal symptoms up to 48 hours before the onset of pain, including fatigue, asthenia, impaired concentration, irritability and other that can warn against an upcoming attack. However, it can be difficult to distinguish prodromal periods in CM as the attacks are very frequent or continuous [24].

Migraine with aura affects 20–40% of all migraineurs [93] and features a selection of transient focal neurological symptoms that usually but not invariably present before the onset of pain. The most common aura type accounting for approximately 90% is visual [84], but patients can also experience sensory, brainstem or hemiplegia-related aura [69, 84, 94]. Both types of migraine, with and without aura, can progress into chronic form.

According to the newest ICHD-3 criteria (**Table 2**), CM should be diagnosed when headache is experienced on 15 or more days per month over more than 3 months. The headache on 8 or more days per month should meet the criteria for migraine with or without aura and/or should be relieved by specific migraine treatment [1].

Not always it is easy for the patients to remember the exact number of days of pain per month, hence keeping a headache diary can come to help. Patients should be encouraged to not only mark the days of pain, but also elaborate what the pain was like, what features it was accompanied by, was any medication required and with what outcome. This is a good and easy tool for a physician to not only accurately know the count up of the headache days, but also make a full picture of its characteristics [95, 96].

Physician making a diagnosis should obtain a detailed history, as history is where the diagnosis of migraine lies. A thorough neurological examination, including fundoscopy, should be the following step during consultation [97].

In case of presentation of typical features of CM and normal examination, no further testing is required. However vigilance is needed to suspect any possible secondary headache causes, such as infections, tumors or hydrocephalus (**Table 3**), when additional investigation is warranted [29]. The set of tests required depends on clinician's judgment in each situation and may include certain blood tests, imaging of brain, cervical spine and sinuses, scanning of cranial and extracranial arteries and performing a lumbar puncture with measuring of the CSF opening pressure. The method of choice for brain imaging is usually MRI [97]. The most consistent indicators for such conditions ("red flags") include thunderclap headache, associated focal neurological deficit or systemic features, headache of onset in patients over the age of 50 years and more [29, 97–99].

After stating that the patient has a primary headache disorder, the pattern of the headache should be established. Episodic headache occurs on less than 15 days per month while chronic headache—on 15 or more days in a month. Headaches lasting up to 4 hours are considered "short" in contrast to "long" headaches that last more

A. Headache (migraine-like or tension-type-like) on ≥15 days/month for >3 months, and fulfilling criteria B and C;
B. Occurring in a patient who has had at least five attacks fulfilling criteria B-D for 1.1 *Migraine without aura* and/or criteria B and C for 1.2 *Migraine with aura*;
C. On ≥8 days/month for >3 months, fulfilling any of the following: 1. Criteria C and D for 1.1 *Migraine without aura*; 2. Criteria B and C for 1.2 *Migraine with aura*; 3. Believed by the patient to be migraine at onset and relieved by a triptan or ergot derivative;
D. Not better accounted for by another ICHD-3 diagnosis.

Table 2.
Chronic migraine diagnostic criteria, ICHD-3, 2018.

Etiology		Examples
Anatomic disorders		Cervical pain, temporomandibular joint disorders, myofascial pain
Changes in intracranial pressure	**Intracranial hypertension**	Tumor, hemorrhage, brain infection, primary benign intracranial hypertension, hydrocephalus, pituitary apoplexy
	Intracranial hypotension	Post-lumbar puncture, post-epidural/spinal analgesia, spontaneous CSF leak
Infection		Meningitis, encephalitis, sinusitis, abscess
Medication and substance disuse		Medication overuse headache, medication side-effects, substance abuse or withdrawal
Metabolic disorders		Uremia, hepatic encephalopathy, hypoxia
Neuralgias		Trigeminal neuralgia, occipital neuralgia
Psychiatric		Somatoform disorder, psychosis, aggravation
Trauma		Traumatic brain injury
Vascular disorders		Stroke, dissection of carotid or vertebral arteries, giant-cell arteritis, arterial hypertension, CADASIL, venous sinuses thrombosis

Table 3.
Possible Causes of Secondary Headaches (alphabetically ordered) [29, 45, 97].

than 4 hours [100]. CM should be differentiated from other chronic long-duration primary headaches (**Table 3**). *Hemicrania continua* is strictly unilateral continuous headache condition with superimposed exacerbations of pain that display ipsilateral autonomic symptoms. CM can also present with autonomic features, but they are much less pronounced. In addition to this, *hemicrania continua* features a distinguishing absolute responsiveness to indomethacin which is a key factor in differential diagnosis [29]. Chronic tension-type headache usually manifests as bilateral ache of non-throbbing quality and mild to moderate severity, while CM can be unilateral or bilateral and of moderate to severe intensity. Importantly, chronic tension-type headache is considered "featureless"—it is not usually accompanied by migrainous symptoms like nausea, vomiting, photophobia, phonophobia, and is not exacerbated by exertion. As migraine progresses into chronic form, the headache may resemble tension-type on some days [29]; nonetheless, typical migraine features must be present on at least 8 days per month for the diagnosis of chronic migraine to be validated [1].

The main feature of new daily persistent headache is a distinct and clearly remembered onset and rapid development to an unremitting state of pain over 24 hours. This distinguishes it from chronic migraine that develops slowly over the course of months or years while attacks become more and more frequent and merged together. Besides, the localization and accompanying symptoms of new daily persistent headache are usually undefined and nonspecific, thus alleviating the differential diagnosis [29, 45, 97].

Another point to remember is the importance of assessing the patient for possible acute medication overuse, as it is one of the major risk factors for migraine progression. Sometimes it may be challenging to tell if medication overuse is a cause or a consequence of CM. The ICHD-3 criteria encourage coding both CM and MOH diagnoses in case when medication overuse is confirmed [1]. The diagnoses should be reviewed and specified later after assessing the effect of medication withdrawal: the headache may revert to episodic migraine or remain chronic. The former case would suggest that medication overuse indeed was a causative factor that had led to chronification. In the latter scenario the diagnosis of medication-overuse headache

Headache type/ causative problem	Localization	Duration	Associated and distinguishing features	Diagnostic tests
Chronic migraine	Unilateral or bilateral	• Hours to days or continuous • Headache present on at least 15 days per month	• Throbbing nature • Accompanying nausea, vomiting, photophobia, phonophobia • Exertional exacerbation	ICH-3 criteria
Hemicrania continua	Side-locked	• Daily, continuous pain with superimposed exacerbations	• Ipsilateral autonomic features • Indomethacin-responsiveness	ICH-3 criteria Indomethacin trial [12]
Chronic tension-type headache	Usually bilateral, but can be unilateral	• Hours to days or continuous	• "Featureless"—no or rare accompanying symptoms	ICH-3 criteria
Medication overuse headache	Undefined	• Hours to days or continuous	• History of acute medication overuse • Improved after withdrawal	ICH-3 criteria
New daily persistent headache	Daily persistent headache with a distinct and clearly remembered onset, with pain becoming continuous and unremitting within 24 hours	Undefined	Undefined	Individual approach: • Brain imaging (CT, MRI) • Lumbar puncture • Blood tests

*Data from Refs. [29, 45, 97].

Table 4.
Differential diagnosis for long-duration primary headaches.*

should be revoked, as it would seem that the overuse had taken place simply as a result of increased attack frequency [101]. Points of the differential diagnosis are summarized in **Table 4**.

Once the diagnosis of CM has been confirmed, standard questionnaires, such as Migraine Disability Assessment (MIDAS) or Headache Impact Test-6 (HIT-6) should be used for patient assessment in order to evaluate the burden of disease and monitor the effects of prescribed treatment [95]. Episodic and treatment-responsive migraine can be diagnosed and managed in the primary care, while chronic or refractory patients should be referred to a specialist neurologist, preferably with an expertise in the field of headache disorders [95].

7. Treatment

There are three broad approaches to treating CM [97]:

- Lifestyle and trigger management.

- Acute headache treatments.
- Preventive treatment.

7.1 Lifestyle and trigger management

Lifestyle modification, as well as trigger reduction can, be helpful in reducing the fequency of migraine attacks and stopping or slowing down the process of migraine chronification. That includes regularity of regimen with regard to meals, hydration, sleep and stress. It could be also helpful to detect and understand the obvious triggers. It is important to know other problems that exacerbate the tendency to headaches: such as: depression, anxiety, other pain syndromes such as fibromyalgia, localized pain in head and neck structures, and conditions that create 'metabolic' strain such as obesity, sleep apnoea or postural orthostatic tachycardia syndrome [102, 103]. It is particularly important to recognize and manage medication overuse (including caffeine overuse), as failure to do so will render most attempts at preventive treatment ineffective [92].

In order to identify the factors mentioned above it is very important to take a detailed history of the particular patient and to evaluate the headache questionnaires and diaries, which are suggestable in many headache centers worldwide.

7.2 Acute headache treatments

The natural course of CM presents a variation in headache frequency meaning that patients can fluctuate between EM and CM [97] and exacerbations of chronic pain. Acute CM treatments are necessary to treat these conditions; e.g., **migraine attacks or exacerbations of chronic pain**.

For the patients with CM often is difficult to know when to take acute treatments. The physician should discuss this question with the patient and also explain about the possibility of co-existence of MOH, which now is considered a sequela rather than a cause of migraine and can co-exist with CM [1, 92].

In order to prevent the development of MOH, it is very important to avoid using painkillers and triptans too often in the early stages of management [104]. The detailed anamnesis and analysis of patient headache questionnaire and diary will help to understand and count the" good days and bad days "or the days with clearly exacerbated headaches. For the acute headache treatment are recommended the same groups of medications as for migraine attack treatment. This includes simple analgesics, combinated analgetics, triptans if the analgetics are not effective, and neuromodulating procedures [97, 99, 105] (Reference to section on treatment of migraine attacks to be included).

Opioids are not recommended for the treatment of acute headache because of the significant risk of medication overuse and the most protracted withdrawal [106].

Triptans are migraine-specific medications that inhibit the release of CGRP by activation of presynaptic 5HT1 receptors [107, 108]. However, patients should not take triptans more than 10 days in a month to avoid developing MOH [1].

Non-invasive stimulation procedures could be used in patients who refuse to use pharmacological migraine therapy or it is contraindicated or not tolerated. That includes external trigeminal nerve stimulation [109], single transcranial magnetic stimulation [110] and transcutaneus vagal nerve stimulation [111].

Effective acute treatment of migraine attacks may help to prevent progression from EM to CM, but rather than relying on taking drugs to stop migraine attacks after they have started, the aim of treatment for CM should be the prevention of migraine attacks [20].

7.3 Preventive treatment

The goals of CM prophylactic treatment are to prevent attacks, thereby reducing headache frequency, severity and associated disability and decreasing reliance on acute treatment, which may be contributing to concurrent MOH [92, 104]. An additional goal may be to prevent progression of EM to CM in patients with high-frequency attacks [45]. The first-line treatment of CM is pharmacological [45].

Numerous orally administered drugs are used for the prophylaxis of CM, including beta-blockers, calcium-channel blockers, tricyclic antidepressants, serotonin antagonists, antihypertensives, and antidepressants [112]. The drugs that are effective for EM are not necessarily effective for CM [54], but evidence for the efficacy of oral agents in CM is generally extrapolated from studies in patients with high-frequency EM [97, 113]. Insufficient efficacy, not suitable route and dose of drug administration and/or adverse events leading to treatment discontinuation often occur with these drugs in patients with CM [114, 115].

The only currently available evidence-based prophylactic treatment options for CM are topiramate and onabotulinumtoxinA (OBT-A) which is a formulation of botulinum toxin A administered by intramuscular injection, from more than one randomized controlled trial [97, 113].

7.3.1 OnabotulinumtoxinA

To date, OBT-A is the only treatment specifically approved for the prevention of CM in the EU and North America (class of evidence I, level of recommendation A) [116–119]. In the Phase III Research Evaluating Migraine Prophylaxis Therapy (PREEMPT) trials [117, 118] OBT-A has been shown to be an effective and generally well tolerated treatment for the prevention of CM, and tends to be better tolerated than various oral prophylactic treatments, including topiramate [120–123]. Based on the PREEMPT clinical trial protocol, OBT-A is administered to at least 31 injection sites across 7 head and neck muscles, and is currently recommended as a second-line option for patients who have not responded adequately or are intolerant of commonly prescribed oral migraine prophylaxis [124]. Treatment should be repeated every 12 weeks. This data was confirmed in recently finished Chronic migraine OnabotulinuMtoxinA Prolonged Efficacy open Label (COMPEL) study, aim to investigate the long-term safety, efficacy and tolerability of nine cycles of repetitive BoNT-A injections. The Compel Study concluded that OBT-A treatment was well tolerated over 108 weeks, and no new safety signals were identified [125].

The molecular biological mechanism of action of OBT-A is well established, whereby it inhibits fusion of intracellular vesicles with the nerve membrane [125] by cleaving synaptosomal-associated protein (SNAP-25) [126, 127]. By impairing intraneuronal vesicular fusion, OBT-A modulates neuropeptide release and downregulates receptors and ion channels important in nociception [128, 129].

So, it is thought that OBT-A blocks release of CGRP from peripheral nociceptive neurons and interferes with transient receptor potential cation (TRP) channels in the trigeminally-innervated cranio-facial-cervical region, thereby reducing neuronal hyperexcitability and peripheral and central sensitisation [54, 130]. It is hypothesized that trigeminal-targeted preventative treatments counteract the impingement of nociceptive input from highly sensitized trigeminal neurons on brainstem second-order neurons, thus preventing central sensitisation, a key pathophysiological mechanism of CM [131].

Additionally recent clinical data demonstrates that OBT-A has been shown to reduce serum CGRP concentration in patients with CM (pretreatment median, 74.1 pg/mL; 1 month post-treatment median, 51.9 pg/mL, $P < 0.001$) [132]. One month after treatment, CGRP levels significantly decreased in patients defined as OBT-A responders.

There is no consensus in the literature regarding the number of OBT-A cycles required for the preventive treatment of CM. Some trials suggest an increasing efficacy with regular cycle repetition for more than 1 year, including in patients with MOH (three class II trials, level B recommendation) [133–135]. To date, no clinical features predicting responses to OBT-A (recommendation level B) have been identified [136, 137].

The adverse effects of this treatment are rare, transient and mild. The most frequently reported were neck and shoulder muscle weakness, post-application headache, palpebral pseudoptosis and other facial mimics asymmetries, in addition to pain at injection sites (class of evidence I) [117–119, 137–139].

7.3.2 Topiramate

Although not specifically licensed for CM, orally administered anticonvulsant topiramate is an effective prophylactic treatment for patients with migraine, and may be effective in patients with CM [140]. Topiramate reduced headache days versus placebo and was relatively well tolerated in patients with CM in two large randomized controlled trials [141, 142]. The initial dosage should be started slowly with 2×12.5 mg or 2×25 mg and a dose of 2×50 mg (if necessary up to 2×100 mg) per day as final target dose. Adverse events commonly associated with topiramate include paresthesia, memory and concentration disturbances, fatigue, nausea, and weight loss [143, 144].

It is thought that topiramate has dual effects on neurotransmission—enhancing inhibitory effects while minimizing excitatory effects, both of which are implicated in migraine physiology [145]. The pharmacologic mechanisms underlying this antimigraine activity may include blockade of cell membrane ion channels and neurotransmitter release (e.g., inhibition of glutamate), resulting in inhibition of neuronal hyperexcitability. Studies have demonstrated topiramate's inhibitory effect on excitability in motor and visual cortices [54, 144, 145]. Based on this broad mechanism of action, topiramate may prevent the development of cortical spreading depression by reducing nociceptive transmission and generally inhibiting neuronal hyperexcitability [146]. Similarly, topiramate has demonstrated cognitive adverse events, which are likely a reflection of the central inhibitory effects [54]. Pooled analyses of clinical trial results suggest that preventive topiramate treatment in patients with episodic migraine may reduce the risk of headache-day increase, which in some cases may prevent migraine chronification [147].

7.3.3 Monoclonal antibodies

Deeper understanding the importance of CGRP and its receptor role in CM pathophysiology and need for more effective, better tolerated prophylactic therapies for CM or high-frequency EM gave background for the development of the new class drugs—anti-CGRP/R monoclonal antibodies (mAbs).

Four anti-CGRP/R antibodies are approved in the US and Europe for the prophylactic treatment of CM: erenumab (Aimovig) [148, 149], which targets the CGRP receptor, fremanezumab (Ajovy) [150, 151] and galcanezumab (Emgality) [152, 153] which target the CGRP ligand; and fourth anti-CGRP/R antibody against the CGRP ligand, eptinezumab (VYEPTI™), which was approved by FDA and EMA on year 2020 [154, 155]. These macromolecule anti-CGRP/R antibodies have been specifically designed for prophylactic use in CM and frequent EM, and to overcome safety issues associated with CGRP receptor antagonists [156, 157]. Eptinezumab

(VYEPTI™) is the first intravenous (IV) treatment for migraine prevention and the latest in a new class of mAbs. A brief review of all four mAbs, dose and rout of adminstration are provided in **Table 5**.

The anti-CGRP/R antibodies are highly specific for their CGRP/R target, have no ability to cross the blood brain barrier, and bypass liver metabolism so CNS-related effects and hepatotoxicity are unlikely [158]. Their long half-lives allow for dosing once a month for erenumab and galcanezumab, or and once every 3 months, for fremanezumab [159–161] and eptinezumab [162].

This very promising treatment with mABs for CM is proved in clinical trials [163].

Erenumab: A phase II RCT evaluated the safety and the efficacy of erenumab in subjects aged 18–65 years with CM with duration of treatment 3 months and preventive treatment not allowed [164]. Patients (n = 667) were randomized to monthly subcutaneous injection of erenumab 70 mg, erenumab 140 mg or placebo for 3 months. Exclusion by preventive failure of >3 drugs. At weeks 9–12, there was a reduction in monthly migraine days in the erenumab 70 mg (LSMD −2.5; SE −3.5 to −1.4; *P* < 0.0001) and in the erenumab 140 mg (LSMD −2.5; SE −3.5 to −1.4; P < 0.0001) groups compared to placebo group. There was a reduction in monthly number of days using migraines-specific medication in the erenumab 70 mg (LSMD −1.9; SE −2.6 to −1.1; P < 0.0001) and in the erenumab 140 mg (LSMD −2.6; SE −3.3 to −1.8; P < 0.0001) groups compared to the placebo group.

Fremanezumab: In this multicentre, randomized, double-blind, double-dummy, placebo-controlled, parallel-group phase 2b study, were enrolled men and

Drug	Manufacturer	Target	Dose of administration	Route of administration	Dosing
Erenumab (Aimovig)	Amgen and Novartis Pharmaceu-ticals	CGRP receptor	70 mg	Once monthly	Autoinjector 70 mg/mL
			140 mg	Some patients may need 140 mg SC once monthly	Autoinjector 140 mg/mL
Fremanezumab (Ajovy)	Teva	CGRP ligand	225 mg	Once monthly	Syringe or autoinjector 225 mg/ 1.5 mL
			675 mg	Every 3 months (q)	
Galcanezumab (Emgality	Eli Lilly and Company	CGRP ligand	240 mg(2 consecutive 120 mg SC injections) loading dose once, maintainance dose 120 mg monthly	Once monthly	Single-dose prefilled pen 120 mg/mL and single-dose prefilled syringe 100 mg/mL and 120 mg/ mL
Eptinezumab (VYEPTI™)	Alder Biopharma-ceuticals and Lundbeck Seattle BioPharma-ceuticals Inc.	CGRP ligand	100 mg IV every 3 months (q)	Every 3 months (q)	Injectable solution 100 mg/ml
			300 mg IV every 3 months (q)	Some patients may benefit from a 300 mg IV dose q3 months	

Table 5.
Brief review of administration of CRRP/R monoclonal antibodies.

women (aged 18–65 years) who had CM with duration of treatment 3 months [165]. Patients (n = 264) were randomized to three 28-day treatment cycles of subcutaneous injections of fremanezumab 225mg, fremanezumab 900mg or placebo. Exclusion by preventive failure of >3 drugs. At weeks 9–12, there was a reduction in moderate to severe headache days in the fremanezumab 675/225mg (LSMD −1.84; 95% CI −3.54 to −0.14; *P* = 0.0345) and in the fremanezumab 900mg (LSMD −1.96; 95% CI −3.66 to −0.26; *P* = 0.0237) groups compared to placebo group. There was a reduction in number of days using acute medication in the fremanezumab 900mg (LSMD −2.04; 95% CI −3.9 to −0.2; *P* = 0.027) group compared to placebo group.

A phase III RCT, the HALO CM, evaluated the efficacy of fremanezumab in subjects aged 18–70years with CM with duration of treatment 3 months [160]. Patients (n = 1130) were randomized to monthly subcutaneous injections of fremanezumab 225mg (loading dose of 675mg), to quarterly fremanezumab 675 mg, or placebo for 3months. Exclusion by preventive failure of ≥2 drugs. During 12-week period, there was a reduction in the average number of headache days per month in the fremanezumab 675mg (LSMD −1.8; SE 0.3; *P* < 0.001) and in the fremanezumab 675/225mg (LSMD -2.1; SE 0.3; P < 0.001) groups compared to placebo group. There was a reduction in the monthly number of days using acute medication in the fremanezumab 675mg (LSMD −1.8; SE 0.3; P < 0.001) and in the fremanezumab 675/225mg (LSMD −2.3; SE 0.3; P < 0.001) groups compared to placebo group. There was an improvement in the HIT-6 [166] score in the fremanezumab 675mg (LSMD −1.9; SE 0.5; P < 0.001) and in the fremanezumab 675/225mg (LSMD −2.4; SE 0.5; P < 0.001) groups compared to placebo group.

Galcanezumab: A phase III RCT, the randomized, double-blind, placebo-controlled REGAIN study evaluated the efficacy of galcanezumab in subjects aged 18–65years with CM with duration of treatment 3 months [161]. Patients (n = 1117) were randomized to monthly subcutaneous injections of galcanezumab 120mg (loading dose of 240mg at baseline), galcanezumab 240mg, or placebo for 3 months. Exclusion by preventive failure of >2 drugs During the 3-month period, there was a reduction in monthly migraine days in the galcanezumab 120mg group (LSMD −2.1; 95% CI −2.9 to −1.3) and with galcanezumab 240mg (LSMD −1.9; 95% CI −2.7 to −1.1) compared to placebo groups. There was a reduction in monthly number of days using acute medication use in the galcanezumab 240mg (LSMD −2.0; 95% CI −2.8 to −1.3) but not in galcanezumab 120mg as compared to the placebo group. There was an improvement in the MIDAS score in the galcanezumab 120mg (LSMD −8.7; 95% CI −16.4 to −3.1) but not in galcanezumab 240mg as compared to the placebo group.

Eptinezumab: This was a phase 2b, parallel-group, double-blind, randomized, placebo-controlled, dose-ranging clinical trial with duration of treatment 12 weeks and preventive treatment, except botulin toxin, not allowed [162]. Men and women aged 18–55 years (n = 616) were included if they had a diagnosis of CM with onset at age 35 years and history of CM 1 year. During the 28-day screening period, patients must have had 15 headache days, including 8 migraine days, with five migraine attacks as recorded in the electronic diary. Exclusion is by preventive failure of ≥2 drugs. Patients were assigned in a 1:1:1:1:1 ratio to eptinezumab 300, 100, 30, 10 mg or placebo, administered as a single IV infusion. The primary endpoint was the percentage of patients with a 75% decrease in monthly migraine days over weeks 1–12 compared with the 28-day screening period. Secondary efficacy endpoints had results favoring the three higher eptinezumab doses versus placebo. The greatest effect of eptinezumab, as measured by the HIT-6 was observed at week 12, with changes in baseline scores of 10.0, 6.9, 6.5, and 6.5 for the 300, 100, 30, and 10 mg groups, respectively, compared with 5.8 for the placebo group. A prespecified analysis of the percentage of patients for whom migraine had a severe impact on life demonstrated a reduction from 90.3% at baseline to 29.9% at week 12 with eptinezumab 300 mg, 86.4–43.0% with eptinezumab 100 mg, compared with 79.3–50.9% with placebo.

The Prevention of Migraine via Intravenous ALD403 Safety and Efficacy–2 (PROMISE-2) study was a phase 3, multicenter, randomized, double-blind, placebo-controlled, parallel-group study with duration of treatment 12 weeks [167]. Adults with CM (n = 1072) were randomly assigned to receive IV eptinezumab 100 mg, eptinezumab 300 mg, or placebo administered on day 0 and week 12. Exclusion is by preventive failure of ≥2 drugs. The primary endpoint was change from baseline in mean monthly migraine days (MMDs) over weeks 1–12. Treatment with eptinezumab 100 and 300 mg was associated with significant reductions in MMDs across weeks 1–12 compared with placebo (placebo −5.6, 100 mg −7.7, $p < 0.0001$ vs. placebo; 300 mg −8.2, $p < 0.0001$ vs. placebo). The mean HIT-6 scores at baseline were 65.0 (eptinezumab 100 mg), 65.1 (eptinezumab 300 mg), and 64.8 (placebo). By week 12, the percentage of patients with HIT-6 scores in the severe range had been reduced to 51.4% in the eptinezumab 100 mg treatment group, 42.9% in the eptinezumab 300 mg treatment group, and 60.1% in the placebo group. Patients in the eptinezumab 300 mg group demonstrated a statistically significant improvement on the HIT-6 at week 12, with an estimated mean difference from placebo (95% confidence interval) of −2.9 (−3.9 to −1.8, $p < 0.0001$).

Adverse events of the mAbs: The results of four mABs clinical studies showed that no serious advers events (SAEs), no deaths deemed to be related to mAbs occurred in clinical trials with all fours mAbs. According the data of clinical trials, the most common adverse events (5 to >10% of the study population) for all three CGRP antagonists (erenumab, fremanezumab, galcanezumab) were injection-site reactions and pain. Specific adverse reactions for erenumab was constipation (1–3% of patients) and cramps, muscle spasms (<3%), hyperintensity for galcanezumab, and nasopharyngitis (6–8%) and hyperintensity (1–2%) for eptinezumab.

Recommendations on the use of the mAbs: Following the clinical studies results and expert opinion EHF on 2019 prepared recommendations about the use three mAbs (erenumab, fremanezumab, galcanezumab) in subjects with CM [163]. In these recommendations due to the then-unpublished original data eptinezumab was not included (**Table 6**). Keeping in mind the fact that this mAb belongs to the same class of drugs (e.g., anti-calcitonin gene-related peptide monoclonal antibodies) with similar profile it seems that the recommendations fits for it too.

7.3.4 Combinations

The strategy of combining different prophylactic drugs is not supported by high-level evidence [168]. However, the so-called rational polytherapy—the association of effective drugs with different mechanisms—can be used in monotherapy-refractory patients [169]. Regarding comparative efficacy, one single-center double-blind RCT showed equivalence between OBT-A (100 units at fixed points plus 100 units at "follow the pain" points) and topiramate (maximum dose of 200 mg), with better tolerability and adherence in the OBT-A [121] while one single-center open-label study showed comparable efficacy between amitriptyline (25–50 mg/day) and OBT-A (250 U/15 sites), also with better tolerability and compliance in the group treated with OBT-A [122].

Preclinical data suggest that anti-calcitonin gene-related peptide monoclonal antibodies and OBT-A have synergistic effects within the trigeminovascular system. Of note, findings indicate that fremanezumab—an antibody targeting the calcitonin

Clinical question	Recommendation	Strength of the recommendation
1. When should treatment with anti-CGRP monoclonal antibodies be offered to patients with migraine?		
	In patients with CM who have failed at least two of the available medical treatments or who cannot use other preventive treatments because of comorbidities, side effects or poor compliance, we suggest the use of erenumab, fremanezumab, or galcanezumab	Experts' opinion
2. How should other preventive treatments be managed when using anti-CGRP monoclonal antibodies in patients with migraine?		
	In patients with CM who are on treatment with any oral drug with inadequate treatment response we suggest to add erenumab, fremanezumab, or galcanezumab and to consider later withdrawal of the oral drug In patients with chronic migraine who are on treatment with OBT-A with inadequate treatment response we suggest to stop OBT-A before initiation of erenumab, fremanezumab, or galcanezumab In patients with CM who are on treatment with erenumab, fremanezumab, or galcanezumab and who may benefit from additional prevention we suggest to add oral preventive drugs	Experts' opinion
3. When should treatment with anti-CGRP monoclonal antibodies be stopped in patients with migraine?		
	In patients with CM, we suggest to consider to stop treatment with erenumab, fremanezumab, and galcanezumab after 6–12 months of treatments	Experts' opinion
4. Should medication overuse be treated before offering treatment anti-CGRP monoclonal antibodies to patients with chronic migraine?		
	In patients with CM and medication overuse, we suggest to use erenumab, fremanezumab, and galcanezumab before or after withdrawal of acute medications	Experts' opinion
5. In which patients anti-CGRP monoclonal antibodies are not to be used?		
	In patients with migraine, we suggest to avoid anti-CGRP monoclonal antibodies in pregnant or nursing women, in individuals with alcohol or drug abuse, cardio and cerebrovascular diseases, and with severe mental disorders	Experts' opinion
6. Should binding and/or neutralizing antibodies be monitored?		
	In patients with migraine on treatment with anti-CGRP monoclonal antibodies, we suggest not to test binding and/or neutralizing antibodies in daily clinical practice; we suggest to further study the possible implications of binding and/or neutralizing antibodies	Experts' opinion

**Adapted with permission: Sacco et al. [163].*

Table 6.
Recommendations on use of anti-calcitonin gene-related peptide monoclonal antibodies in subjects with chronic migraine.*

gene-related peptide—mainly prevents the activation of Aδ-fibers, whereas botulinum toxin type A prevents the activation of C-fibers [168]. There is currently only indirect preclinical evidence to support a rationale for dual therapy with anti-calcitonin gene-related peptide monoclonal antibodies and OBT-A for CM prevention [170]. Rigorous studies evaluating clinical efficacy, safety, and cost-effectiveness of dual therapy with mAbs are needed.

8. Management of chronic migraine

CM is underdiagnosed and, thus, untreated disease. Only 20% of patients who meet the criteria for CM are properly diagnosed [65].Treatment options are available for these patients, but only if the patients are properly identified [171]. Successful management of CM will help properly diagnose this disease, optimize treatment and thus reduce the global burden of it. Important components of CM management involve correct diagnosis, optimal treatment plan, patient education, treatment of MOH and comorbid conditions and monitoring of patients response to treatment plan.

It is important for all physicians who are treating the patient to understand the treatment plan, in order to monitor the patient's response to treatment, using as well as continual assessment of the patient's Health-Related Quality of Life (HRQOL) [95]. Preventive therapy for migraines may take up to 6–8 weeks to begin to demonstrate efficacy, and up to 6 months before full efficacy is established [172]. Support and close follow-up are essential for patients, particularly in the first 3 months of treatment [172].

Additionally, physicians should try to identify and reduce aggravating risk factors, such as triggers of migraine or other behavioral habits that may have contributed to the patient's headaches (Section 7.1).

Thus, multimodal treatment concepts are superior to simple drug treatment in severely affected patients [95].

Box 1 contains the key components of chronic migraine management for physicians [95].

Complete and correct diagnosis
Referral to headache specialist/neurologist to confirm CM diagnosis and provide a treatment plan
Management of overuse of acute headache pain medications: providing limits to acute and rescue therapy
Patient education about CM and importance of treatment compliance
Explaining realistic expectations to patients
Consideration of important exacerbating factors
Treatment of comorbid conditions
Nonpharmacotherapy, including trigger management and behavioral therapy
CM, chronic migraine; HIT-6, headache impact test-6; HRQoL, health-related quality of life; MIDAS, migraine disability assessment.

*With permission: Diener et al. [95].

Box 1.
*Important components of chronic migraine management**.

9. Conclusions

CM is associated with higher burden of disease, more severe psychiatric comorbidity, greater use of healthcare resources, and higher total costs than EM. The current definition of CM has gone through multiple revisions, but the discussion about it is still continuing,

The pathophysiology of CM is not fully understood. However, recent advances in electrophysiology and neuroimaging have indicated that atypical pain processing, central sensitization, cortical hyperexcitability and neurogenic inflammation are important in the development of this disorder. The most significant risk factors such as overuse of acute medication, ineffective acute treatment, obesity, depression and stressful life events have been associated with migraine progression.

Unfortunately, CM is still undertreated because of its poor treatment response and limited therapy options. The currently available evidence-based prophylactic treatment options for CM are topiramate and OBT-A. According to the results of the clinical studies the new class of drugs—anti-CGRP/R monoclonal antibodies seems to be a very promising treatment for CM. Complete and correct diagnosis, optimal treatment plan, management of acute medication overuse and exacerbating factors, patient education and monitoring of the patient's response to treatment plan are the most important components for the successful CM management.

The next years seem to be inspiring for the field, as current research areas are being extended and novel areas are being covered, ultimately broadening our understanding of the complex syndrome of CM.

Conflict of interest

The authors declare that they have no conflict of interest related to the publication of this chapter.

Abbreviations

CM	chronic migraine
HIS	the International Headache Society
EM	episodic migraine
MIDAS	Migraine Disability Assessment
ICHD-3	International Classification of Headache Disorders, 3rd edition
ICHD-1	International Classification of Headache Disorders, 1st edition
ICHD-2	Classification of Headache Disorders, 2nd edition
MOH	medication-overuse headache
CSD	cortical spreading depression
VIP	vasoactive intestinal peptide
CGRP	calcitonin gene-related peptide
HIT-6	Headache Impact Test-6
5HT1	serotonin 1a
OBT-A	onabotulinumtoxinA
FDA	U.S. Food & Drug Administration
EMA	European Medicines Agency
HRQoL	health-related quality of life

Author details

Diana Obelieniene[1*], Ruta Pestininkaite[2] and Daiva Rastenyte[2]

1 Department of Neurology, Hospital of Lithuanian University of Health Sciences (LSMU) Kauno Klinikos, Kaunas, Lithuania

2 Department of Neurology, Medical Academy, Lithuanian University of Health Sciences (LSMU), Kaunas, Lithuania

*Address all correspondence to: diana.obelieniene@kaunoklinikos.lt

References

[1] Headache Classification Committee of the International Headache Society (IHS). The International Classification of Headache Disorders ICHD-3, 3rd edition. Cephalalgia. 2018;**38**(1): 1-211

[2] Buse DC et al. Chronic migraine prevalence, disability, and sociodemographic factors: Results from the American Migraine Prevalence and Prevention Study. Headache. 2012;**52**: 1456-1470

[3] Blumenfeld AM et al. Disability, HRQoL and resource use among chronic and episodic migraineurs: Results from the International Burden of Migraine Study (IBMS). Cephalalgia. 2011;**31**: 301-315

[4] Wiendels NJ et al. Chronic frequent headache in the general population: Comorbidity and quality of life. Cephalalgia. 2006;**26**:1443-1450

[5] Berra E et al. Cost of chronic and episodic migraine. A pilot study from tertiary headache centre northern Italy. The Journal of Headache and Pain. 2015; **16**:532

[6] Munakata J et al. Economic burden of transformed migraine: results from the American Migraine Prevalence and Prevention (AMPP) Study. Headache. 2009;**49**:498-508

[7] Magiorkinis E, Diamantis A, Mitsikostas DD, Androutsos G. Headaches in antiquity and during the early scientific era. Journal of Neurology. 2009;**256**:1215-1220

[8] Ad Hoc Committee on Classification of Headache. Classification of headache. JAMA. 1962;**179**:717-718

[9] Headache Classification Committee of the International Headache Society. Classification and diagnostic criteria for headache disorders, cranial neuralgias and facial pain. Cephalalgia. 1988;**8**:1-96

[10] Manack A, Turkel C, Silberstein S. The evolution of chronic migraine: Classification and nomenclature. Headache. 2009;**49**:1206-1213

[11] Mathew NT, Stubits E, Nigam MP. Transformation of episodic migraine into daily headache: Analysis of factors. Headache. 1982;**22**:66-68

[12] Mathew NT, Reuveni U, Perez F. Transformed or evolutive migraine. Headache. 1987;**27**:102-106

[13] Silberstein SD, Lipton RB, Solomon SMN. Classification of daily and near daily headaches: Proposed revisions to the IHS criteria. Headache. 1994;**34**:1-7

[14] Silberstein SD, Lipton RB, Sliwinski M. Classification of daily and near-daily headaches: Field trial of revised IHS criteria. Neurology. 1996; **47**:871-875

[15] Manzoni GC, Granella F, Sandrini G, Cavallini A, Zanferrari C, Nappi G. Classification of chronic daily headache by International Headache Society criteria: Limits and new proposals. Cephalalgia. 1995;**15**:37-43

[16] Headache Classification Subcommittee of the International Headache Society. The International Classification of Headache Disorders. Cephalalgia. 2004;**24**:1-160

[17] Medrea I, Christie S. Evolution of the concept and clinical implications. Headache. 2018;**58**:1495-1500

[18] Bigal ME, Tepper SJ, Sheftell FD, Rapoport AM, Lipton RB. Chronic daily headache: Correlation between the 2004 and the 1988 International Headache

Society diagnostic criteria. Headache. 2004;**44**:684-691

[19] Chalmer MA, Hansen TF, Lebedeva ER, et al. Proposed new diagnostic criteria for chronic migraine. Cephalalgia. 2020;**40**(4):399-406. DOI: 10.1177/0333102419877171

[20] Natoli JL, Manack A, Dean B, Butler Q, Turkel CC, Stovner L, et al. Global prevalence of chronic migraine: A systematic review. Cephalalgia. 2010; **30**(5):599-609

[21] Katsarava Z et al. Primary headache disorders in the Republic of Georgia Prevalence and risk factors. Neurology. 2009;**73**:1796-1803

[22] Scher AI, Stewart WF, Liberman J, Lipton RB. Prevalence of frequent headache in a population sample. Headache. 1998;**38**:497-506

[23] Yoon MS et al. Prevalence of primary headaches in Germany: Results of the German Headache Consortium Study. The Journal of Headache and Pain. 2012;**13**:215-223

[24] Katsarava Z, Buse DC, Manack AN, Lipton RB. Defining the differences between episodic migraine and chronic migraine. Current Pain and Headache Reports. 2012;**16**(1):86-92

[25] Buse DC, Manack A, Serrano D, Turkel C, Lipton RB. Sociodemographic and comorbidity profiles of chronic migraine and episodic migraine sufferers. Journal of Neurology, Neurosurgery, and Psychiatry. 2010;**81**: 428-432

[26] Buse DC, Greisman JD, Baigi K, Lipton RB. Migraine progression: A systematic review. Headache. 2019; **59**(3):306-338

[27] Scher AI, Stewart WF, Ricci JA, Lipton RB. Factors associated with the onset and remission of chronic daily headache in a population-based study. Pain. 2003;**106**:81-89

[28] Goadsby PJ, Holland PR, Martinsoliveira M, Hoffmann J, Schankin C, Akerman S. Pathophysiology of migraine: A disorder of sensory processing. Physiological Reviews. 2017;**97**:553-622

[29] Schwedt TJ. Chronic migraine. BMJ. 2014;**348**:g1416. DOI: 10.1136/bmj.g1416

[30] Goadsby PJ. Migraine, aura and cortical spreading depression: Why are we still talking about it? Annals of Neurology. 2001;**49**:4-6. [PubMed: 11198295]

[31] McNaughton FL, Feindel WH. Innervation of intracranial structures: A reappraisal. In: Rose FC, editor. Physiological Aspects of Clinical Neurology. Oxford: Blackwell Scientific; 1977. pp. 279-293

[32] Penfield W, McNaughton FL. Dural headache and the innervation of the dura mater. Archives of Neurology and Psychiatry. 1940;**44**:43-75

[33] Ray BS, Wolff HG. Experimental studies on headache. Pain sensitive structures of the head and their significance in headache. Archives of Surgery. 1940;**41**:813-856

[34] Marfurt CF. The central projections of trigeminal primary afferent neurons in the cat as determined by the tranganglionic transport of horseradish peroxidase. The Journal of Comparative Neurology. 1981;**203**:785-798. [PubMed: 6173403]

[35] Goadsby PJ, Hoskin KL. The distribution of trigeminovascular afferents in the nonhuman primate brain *Macaca nemestrina*: A c-fos immunocytochemical study. Journal of Anatomy. 1997;**190**:367-375. [PMCID: PMC1467617] [PubMed: 9147223]

[36] Hoskin KL, Zagami A, Goadsby PJ. Stimulation of the middle meningeal artery leads to expression in the trigeminocervical nucleus: A comparative study of monkey and cat. Journal of Anatomy. 1999;**194**:579-588. [PMCID: PMC1467956] [PubMed: 10445825]

[37] SWG D, AKP J, Gyulai F, Clark S, Townsend D, Firestone LL. Pain processing during three levels of noxious stimulation produces differential patterns of central activity. Pain. 1997;**73**:431-445. [PubMed: 9469535]

[38] Burstein R, Jakubowski M. Neural substrate of depression during migraine. Neurological Sciences. 2009;**30**(Suppl 1): S27-S31. [PubMed: 19415422]

[39] Kunkler PE, Kraig RP. Cortical spreading depression bilaterally activates the caudal trigeminal nucleus in rodents. Hippocampus. 2003;**13**: 835-844. [PMCID: PMC2805270] [PubMed: 14620879]

[40] Moulton EA, Burstein R, Tully S, Hargreaves R, Becerra L, Borsook D. Interictal dysfunction of a brainstem descending modulatory center in migraine patients. PLoS One. 2008;**3**: e3799

[41] Schwedt TJ, Larson-Prior L, Coalson RS, Nolan T, Mar S, Ances BM, et al. Allodynia and descending pain modulation in migraine: A resting state functional connectivity analysis. Pain Medicine. 2014;**15**:154-165

[42] Aurora SK, Barrodale PM, Tipton RL, Khodavirdi A. Brainstem dysfunction in chronic migraine as evidenced byneurophysiological and positron emission tomography studies. Headache. 2007;**47**:996-1003; discussion 1004-7

[43] Lai TH, Chou KH, Fuh JL, et al. Gray matter changes related to medication overuse in patients with chronic migraine. Cephalalgia. 2016;**36** (14):1324-1333. DOI: 10.1177/0333102416630593

[44] Heinricher MM, Tavares I, Leith JL, Lumb BM. Descending control of nociception: Specificity, recruitment and plasticity. Brain Research Reviews. 2009;**60**:214-225

[45] May A, Schulte LH. Chronic migraine: Risk factors, mechanisms and treatment. Nature Reviews. Neurology. 2016;**12**(8):455-464. DOI: 10.1038/nrneurol.2016.93

[46] Stankewitz A, Aderjan D, Eippert F, May A. Trigeminal nociceptive transmission in migraineurs predicts migraine attacks. The Journal of Neuroscience. 2011;**31**(6):1937-1943. DOI: 10.1523/4496-10.2011

[47] Schulte LH, Jürgens TP, May A. Photo-, osmo- and phonophobia in the premonitory phase of migraine: Mistaking symptoms for triggers? The Journal of Headache and Pain. 2015;**16**: 14. DOI: 10.1186/s10194-015-0495-7

[48] Dahlem MA, Kurths J, Ferrari MD, Aihara K, Scheffer M, May A. Understanding migraine using dynamic network biomarkers. Cephalalgia. 2015; **35**(7):627-630. DOI: 10.1177/0333102414550108

[49] Katsarava Z, Schneeweiss S, Kurth T, et al. Incidence and predictors for chronicity of headache in patients with episodic migraine. Neurology. 2004;**62**(5):788-790. DOI: 10.1212/01.wnl.0000113747.18760.d2

[50] Louter MA, Bosker JE, Van Oosterhout WPJ, Van Zwet EW, Zitman FG, Ferrari MD, et al. Cutaneous allodynia as a predictor of migraine chronification. Brain. 2013; **136**(11):3489-3496

[51] Lipton RB, Fanning KM, Serrano D, Reed ML, Cady R, Buse DC. Ineffective

acute treatment of episodic migraine is associated with new-onset chronic migraine. Neurology. 2015;**84**(7): 688-695

[52] Burstein R. Deconstructing migraine headache into peripheral and central sensitization. Pain. 2001;**89**(2–3): 107-110

[53] Mathew NT, Kurman R, Perez F. Drug induced refractory headache—Clinical features and management. Headache. 1990;**30**(10):634-638. DOI: 10.1111/j.1526-4610.1990.hed3010634.x

[54] Aurora SK, Brin MF. Chronic migraine: An update on physiology, imaging, and the mechanism of action of two available pharmacologic therapies. Headache. 2017;**57**(1): 109-125. DOI: 10.1111/head.12999

[55] Su M, Yu S. Chronic migraine: A process of dysmodulation and sensitization. Molecular Pain. 2018;**14**: 1744806918767697. DOI: 10.1177/1744806918767697

[56] Ramachandran R. Neurogenic inflammation and its role in migraine. Seminars in Immunopathology. 2018; **40**(3):301-314. DOI: 10.1007/s00281-018-0676-y

[57] Cernuda-Morollón E, Martínez-Camblor P, Ramón C, Larrosa D, Serrano-Pertierra E, Pascual J. CGRP and VIP levels as predictors of efficacy of onabotulinumtoxin type a in chronic migraine. Headache. 2014;**54**(6): 987-995

[58] Cernuda-Morollon E, Martinez-Camblor P, Alvarez R, Larrosa D, Ramon C, Pascual J. Increased VIP levels in peripheral blood outside migraine attacks as a potential biomarker of cranial parasympathetic activation in chronic migraine. Cephalalgia. 2015; **35**(4):310-316

[59] Cernuda-Morollón E, Larrosa D, Ramón C, Vega J, Martínez-Camblor P, Pascual J. Interictal increase of CGRP levels in peripheral blood as a biomarker for chronic migraine. Neurology. 2013; **81**(14):1191-1196. DOI: 10.1212/WNL.0b013e3182a6cb72

[60] Ramón C, Cernuda-Morollón E, Pascual J. Calcitonin gene-related peptide in peripheral blood as a biomarker for migraine. Current Opinion in Neurology. 2017;**30**(3): 281-286. DOI: 10.1097/WCO.0000000000000440

[61] Toghae M, Rahimian E, Abdollahi M, Shoar S, Naderan M. The prevalence of magnetic resonance imaging hyperintensity in migraine patients and its association with migraine headache characteristics and cardiovascular risk factors. Oman Medical Journal. 2015;**30**(3):203-207

[62] Maleki N, Becerra L, Brawn J, Bigal M, Burstein R, Borsook D. Concurrent functional and structural cortical alterations in migraine. Cephalalgia. 2012;**32**(8):607-620

[63] Magon S, May A, Stankewitz A, Goadsby PJ, Schankin C, Ashina M, et al. Cortical abnormalities in episodic migraine: a multi-center 3T MRI study. Cephalalgia. 2019;**39**(5):665-673

[64] Torres-Ferrús M, Ursitti F, Alpuente-Ruiz A, et al. From transformation to chronification of migraine: Pathophysiological and clinical aspects. The Journal of Headache and Pain. 2020;**21**(1):42. DOI: 10.1186/s10194-020-01111-8

[65] Bigal ME, Serrano D, Reed M, Lipton RB. Chronic migraine in the spopulation: burden, diagnosis, and satisfaction with treatment. Neurology. 2008;**71**(8):559-566

[66] Goldman D, Oroszi G, Ducci F. The genetics of addictions: Uncovering the genes. Nature Reviews. Genetics. 2005; **6**(7):521-532

[67] Vila-Pueyo M, Fernandez-Castillo N, Cormand B, Pozo-Rosich P, Macaya A. Epigenetic changes in a rat model of migraine with aura. The Journal of Headache and Pain. 2014;**15** (Suppl 1):A6. DOI: 10.1186/1129-2377-15-S1-A6

[68] Nelson ED, Monteggia LM. Epigenetics in the mature mammalian brain: Effects on behavior and synaptic transmission. Neurobiology of Learning and Memory. 2011;**96**(1):53-60

[69] Bigal ME, Lipton RB. Migraine chronification. Current Neurology and Neuroscience Reports. 2011;**11**(2): 139-148

[70] Stewart WF, Lipton RB, Dowson AJ, Sawyer J. Development and testing of the Migraine Disability Assessment (MIDAS) Questionnaire to assess headache-related disability. Neurology. 2001;**56**(suppl 1):S20 LP-S20S28

[71] Bigal ME, Lipton RB. Obesity and chronic daily headache. Current Pain and Headache Reports. 2008;**12**(1): 56-61

[72] Ashina S, Serrano D, Lipton RB, et al. Depression and risk of transformation of episodic to chronic migraine. The Journal of Headache and Pain. 2012;**13**(8):615-624. DOI: 10.1007/s10194-012-0479-9

[73] Finocchi C, Strada L. Sex-related differences in migraine. Neurological Sciences. 2014;**35**(Suppl 1):207-213

[74] Lipton RB, Stewart WF, Diamond S, Diamond ML, Reed M. Prevalence and burden of migraine in the United States: Data from the American migraine study II. Headache. 2001;**41**(7):646-657

[75] Adams AM, Serrano D, Buse DC, et al. The impact of chronic migraine: The Chronic Migraine Epidemiology and Outcomes (CaMEO) Study methods and baseline results. Cephalalgia. 2015;**35**(7): 563-578. DOI: 10.1177/0333102414552532

[76] Lu S-R, Fuh J-L, Wang S-J, Juang K-D, Chen S-P, Liao Y-C, et al. Incidence and risk factors of chronic daily headache in young adolescents: A school cohort study. Pediatrics. 2013;**132**(1):e9-e16

[77] Scher AI, Stewart WF, Lipton RB. Caffeine as a risk factor for chronic daily headache: A population-based study. Neurology. 2004;**63**(11):2022-2027

[78] Santos IS, Goulart AC, Passos VM, del Carmen MM, Lotufo PA, Bensenor IM. Obesity, abdominal obesity and migraine: A crosssectional analysis of ELSA-Brasil baseline data. Cephalalgia. 2015;**35**(5):426-436

[79] Ornello R, Ripa P, Pistoia F, Degan D, Tiseo C, Carolei A, et al. Migraine and body mass index categories: A systematic review and meta-analysis of observational studies. The Journal of Headache and Pain. 2015;**16**:27

[80] Fava A, Pirritano D, Consoli D, et al. Chronic migraine in women is associated with insulin resistance: A cross-sectional study. European Journal of Neurology. 2014;**21**(2):267-272. DOI: 10.1111/ene.12289

[81] Peterlin BL, Rosso AL, Rapoport AM, Scher AI. Obesity and migraine: The effect of age, gender and adipose tissue distribution. Headache. 2010;**50**(1):52-62. DOI: 10.1111/j.1526-4610.2009.01459.x

[82] He Z, Dong L, Zhang Y, Kong Q, Tan G, Zhou J. Metabolic syndrome in female migraine patients is associated with medication overuse headache: A clinic-based study in China. European Journal of Neurology. 2015;**22**(8): 1228-1234. DOI: 10.1111/ene.12732

[83] Buse DC, Rains JC, Pavlovic JM, Fanning KM, Reed ML, Manack

Adams A, et al. Sleep disorders among people with migraine: Results from the chronic migraine epidemiology and outcomes (CaMEO) study. Headache. 2019;**59**(1):32-45

[84] Bigal ME, Lipton RB. What predicts the change from episodic tochronic migraine? Current Opinion in Neurology. 2009;**22**(3):269-276

[85] Lipton RB, Fanning KM, Buse DC, Martin VT, Hohaia LB, Adams AM, et al. Migraine progression in subgroups of migraine based on comorbidities: Results of the CaMEO study. Neurology. 2019;**93**(24):e2224-e2236

[86] Buse D, Silberstein S, Manack A, Papapetropoulos S, Lipton R. Psychiatric comorbidities of episodic and chronic migraine. Journal of Neurology. 2013;**260**(8):1960-1969

[87] Kayhan F, Ilik F. Prevalence of personality disorders in patients with chronic migraine. Comprehensive Psychiatry. 2016;**68**:60-64

[88] Plesh O, Adams SH, Gansky SA. Self-reported comorbid pains in severe headaches or migraines in a US national sample. Headache. 2012;**52**(6):946-956

[89] Lipton RB, Bigal ME, Ashina S, Burstein R, Silberstein S, Reed ML, et al. Cutaneous allodynia in the migraine population. Annals of Neurology. 2008; **63**(2):148-158

[90] Lampl C, Huber G, Haas S, Rittberger E, Diener HC. Difference in triptan effect in patients with migraine and early allodynia. Cephalalgia. 2008; **28**(10):1031-1038

[91] Kristoffersen ES, Grande RB, Aaseth K, Russell MB, Lundqvist C. Medication-overuse headache detoxification reduces headache disability—The Akershus study of chronic headache. European Journal of Neurology. 2018;**25**(9):1140-1147

[92] Ferrari A, Baraldi C, Sternieri E. Medication overuse and chronic migraine: A critical review according to clinical pharmacology. Expert Opinion on Drug Metabolism & Toxicology. 2015;**11**(7):1127-1144

[93] Buse DC, Loder EW, Gorman JA, et al. Sex differences in the prevalence, symptoms, and associated features of migraine, probable migraine and other severe headache: Results of the American Migraine Prevalence and Prevention (AMPP) Study. Headache. 2013;**53**(8): 1278-1299. DOI: 10.1111/head.12150

[94] Russell MB, Ducros A. Sporadic and familial hemiplegic migraine: Pathophysiological mechanisms, clinical characteristics, diagnosis, and management. Lancet Neurology. 2011; **10**(5):457-470. DOI: 10.1016/S1474 4422(11)70048-5

[95] Diener HC, Solbach K, Holle D, Gaul C. Integrated care for chronic migraine patients: Epidemiology, burden, diagnosis and treatment options. Clinical Medicine (London, England). 2015;**15**(4):344-350. DOI: 10.7861/clinmedicine.15-4-344

[96] Dodick DW, Silberstein SD. Migraine prevention. Practical Neurology. 2007;**7**:383-393

[97] Weatherall MW. The diagnosis and treatment of chronic migraine. Therapeutic Advances in Chronic Diseases. 2015;**6**(3):115-123. DOI: 10.1177/2040622315579627

[98] Yancey JR, Sheridan R, Koren KG. Chronic daily headache: Diagnosis and management. American Family Physician. 2014;**89**(8):642-648

[99] British Association for the Study of Headache (BASH). National Headache Management System for Adults Guidelines. 2019. Available from: www.bash.org.uk

[100] Welch KM, Goadsby PJ. Chronic daily headache: Nosology and pathophysiology. Current Opinion in Neurology. 2002;**15**(3):287-295. DOI: 10.1097/00019052-200206000-00011

[101] Viana M, Bottiroli S, Sances G, et al. Factors associated to chronic migraine with medication overuse: A cross-sectional study. Cephalalgia. 2018; **38**(14):2045-2057. DOI: 10.1177/0333102418761047

[102] Serrano D, Lipton RB, Scher AI, Reed ML, Stewart WBF, Adams AM, et al. Fluctuations in episodic and chronic migraine status over the course of 1 year: Implications for diagnosis, treatment and clinical trial design. The Journal of Headache and Pain. 2017; **18**(1):101

[103] Bigal ME, Lipton RB. Modifiable risk factors for migraine progression. Headache. 2006;**46**(9):1334-1343

[104] Limmroth V, Katsarava Z, Fritsche G, Przywara S, Diener HC. Features of medication overuse headache following overuse of different acute headache drugs. Neurology. 2002; **59**(7):1011-1014

[105] Diener HC, Holle-Lee D, Nägel S, Gaul C. Differenzialtherapie von Kopfschmerzen [Headache Treatment]. Dtsch Med Wochenschr. 2017;**142**(6): 418-426. DOI: 10.1055/s-0042-121336

[106] Totzeck A, Gaul C. The role of opioids in the treatment of primary headache disorders. Schmerz. 2014; **28**(2):135-140

[107] Dussor G, Yan J, Xie JY, Ossipov MH, Dodick DW, Porreca F. Targeting TRP channels for novel migraine therapeutics. ACS Chemical Neuroscience. 2014;**5**(11):1085-1096

[108] Ho TW, Edvinsson L, Goadsby PJ. CGRP and its receptors provide new insights into migraine pathophysiology. Nature Reviews. Neurology. 2010; **6**(10):573-582

[109] Schoenen J, Vandersmissen B, Jeangette S, et al. Migraine prevention with a supraorbital transcutaneous stimulator: A randomized controlled trial. Neurology. 2013;**80**(8):697-704

[110] Lipton RB, Dodick DW, Silberstein SD, et al. Single-pulse transcranial magnetic stimulation for acute treatment of migraine with aura: A randomised, double-blind, parallel-group, shamcontrolled trial. Lancet Neurology. 2010;**9**(4):373-380

[111] Silberstein SD, Calhoun AH, Lipton RB, et al. Chronic migraine headache prevention with noninvasive vagus nerve stimulation: The EVENT study. Neurology. 2016;**87**(5):529-538

[112] Sarchielli P, Granella F, Prudenzano MP, Pini LA, Guidetti V, Bono G, et al. Italian guidelines for primary headaches: 2012 revised version. The Journal of Headache and Pain. 2012;**13**(Suppl 2):S31-S70

[113] Cho SJ, Song TJ, Chu MK. Treatment update of chronic migraine. Current Pain and Headache Reports. 2017;**21**(6):26

[114] Hepp Z, Bloudek LM, Varon SF. Systematic review of migraine prophylaxis adherence and persistence. Journal of Managed Care Pharmacy. 2014;**20**(1):22-33

[115] Hepp Z, Dodick DW, Varon SF, Gillard P, Hansen RN, Devine EB. Adherence to oral migraine-preventive medications among patients with chronic migraine. Cephalalgia. 2015; **35**(6):478-488

[116] BOTOX (OnabotulinumtoxinA for Injection, for Intramuscular, Intradetrusor, or Intradermal Use). Irvine, CA: Full Prescribing Information, Allergan, Inc; 2013

[117] Aurora SK, Dodick DW, Turkel CC, DeGryse RE, Silberstein SD, Lipton RB, et al. Onabotulinumtoxin A for treatment of chronic migraine: results from the double-blind, randomized, placebo-controlled phase of the PREEMPT 1 trial. Cephalalgia. 2010;**30**(7):793-803

[118] Diener HC, Dodick DW, Aurora SK, Turkel CC, DeGryse RE, Lipton RB, et al. OnabotulinumtoxinA for treatment of chronic migraine: Results from the double-blind, randomized, placebo-controlled phase of the PREEMPT 2 trial. Cephalalgia. 2010;**30**(7):804-814

[119] Dodick DW, Turkel CC, DeGryse RE, Aurora SK, Silberstein SD, Lipton RB, et al. OnabotulinumtoxinA for treatment of chronic migraine: Pooled results from the double-blind, randomized, placebo-controlled phases of the PREEMPT clinical program. Headache. 2010;**50**(6):921-936

[120] Blumenfeld AM, Schim JD, Chippendale TJ. Botulinum toxin type a and divalproex sodium for prophylactic treatment of episodic or chronic migraine. Headache. 2008;**48**(2): 210-220

[121] Mathew NT, Jaffri SF. A double-blind comparison of onabotulinumtoxinA (BOTOX) and topiramate (TOPAMAX) for the prophylactic treatment of chronic migraine: a pilot study. Headache. 2009; **49**(10):1466-1478

[122] Magalhaes E, Menezes C, Cardeal M, Melo A. Botulinum toxin type a versus amitriptyline for the treatment of chronic daily migraine. Clinical Neurology and Neurosurgery. 2010;**112**(6):463-466

[123] Tassorelli C, Aguggia M, De Tommaso M, Geppetti P, Grazzi L, Pini LA, et al. Onabotulinumtoxin a for the management of chronic migraine in current clinical practice: Results of a survey of sixty-three Italian headache centers. The Journal of Headache and Pain. 2017;**18**(1):66

[124] Tassorelli C, Tedeschi G, Sarchielli P, Pini LA, Grazzi L, Geppetti P, et al. Optimizing the long-term management of chronic migraine with onabotulinumtoxinA in real life. Expert Review of Neurotherapeutics. 2018;**18**(2):167-176

[125] Winner PK, Blumenfield AM, Eross EJ, et al. Long-term safety and tolerability of onabotulinumtoxinA treatment in patients with chronic migraine: Results of the COMPEL study. Drug Safety. 2019;**42**(8):1013-1024

[126] Simpson LL. The origin, structure, and pharmacological activity of botulinum toxin. Pharmacological Reviews. 1981;**33**:155-188

[127] Blasi J, Chapman ER, Link E, et al. Botulinum neurotoxin A selectively cleaves the synaptic protein SNAP-25. Nature. 1993;**365**:160-163

[128] Burstein R, Zhang X, Levy D, Aoki KR, Brin MF. Selective inhibition of meningeal nociceptors by botulinum neurotoxin type A: Therapeutic implications for migraine and other pains. Cephalalgia. 2014;**34**:853-869

[129] Whitcup SM, Turkel CC, DeGryse RE, Brin MF. Development of onabotulinumtoxinA for chronic migraine. Annals of the New York Academy of Sciences. 2014;**1329**:67-80

[130] Frampton JE, Silberstein S. OnabotulinumtoxinA: A review in the prevention of chronic migraine. Drugs. 2018;**78**(5):589-600

[131] Agostoni EC, Barbanti P, Calabresi P, et al. Current and emerging evidence-based treatment options in chronic migraine: A narrative review. The Journal of Headache and Pain. 2019;**20**:92

[132] Cernuda-Morollon E, Ramon C, Martinez-Camblor P, Serrano-Pertierra E, Larrosa D, Pascual J. OnabotulinumtoxinA decreases interictal CGRP plasma levels in patients with chronic migraine. Pain. 2015;**156**: 820-824

[133] Guerzoni S, Pellesi L, Baraldi C, Pini LA. Increased efficacy of regularly repeated cycles with onabotulinumtoxinA in MOH patients beyond the first year of treatment. The Journal of Headache and Pain. 2015;**17**:48

[134] Silberstein SD, Dodick DW, Aurora SK, Diener HC, DeGryse RE, Lipton RB, et al. Per cent of patients with chronic migraine who responded per onabotulinumtoxinA treatment cycle: PREEMPT. Journal of Neurology, Neurosurgery, and Psychiatry. 2015; **86**(9):996-1001

[135] Sarchielli P, Romoli M, Corbelli I, Bernetti L, Verzina A, Brahimi E, et al. Stopping onabotulinum treatment after the first two cycles might not be justified: Results of a real-life monocentric prospective study in chronic migraine. Frontiers in Neurology. 2017;**8**:655

[136] Barbanti P, Ferroni P. Onabotulinum toxin A in the treatment of chronic migraine: Patient selection and special considerations. Journal of Pain Research. 2017;**10**:2319-2329

[137] Blumenfeld AM, Stark RJ, Freeman MC, Orejudos A, Manack AA. Long-term study of the efficacy and safety of onabotulinumtoxinA for the prevention of chronic migraine: COMPEL study. The Journal of Headache and Pain. 2018;**19**(1):13

[138] Matharu M, Pascual J, Nilsson Remahl I, Straube A, Lum A, Davar G, et al. Utilization and safety of onabotulinumtoxinA for the prophylactic treatment of chronic migraine from an observational study in Europe. Cephalalgia. 2017;**37**(14):1384-1397

[139] Bendtsen L, Sacco S, Ashina M, Mitsikostas D, Ahmed F, Pozo-Rosich P, et al. Guideline on the use of onabotulinumtoxinA in chronic migraine: A consensus statement from the European Headache Federation. The Journal of Headache and Pain. 2018;**19**(1):91

[140] Cady RK, Schreiber CP, Porter JA, Blumenfeld AM, Farmer KU. A multi-center double-blind pilot comparison of onabotulinumtoxinA and topiramate for the prophylactic treatment of chronic migraine. Headache. 2011;**51**:21-32

[141] Diener HC, Bussone G, Van Oene JC, Lahaye M, Schwalen S, Goadsby PJ. Topiramate reduces headache days in chronic migraine: a randomized, double-blind, placebo-controlled study. Cephalalgia. 2007; **27**(7):814-823

[142] Silberstein SD, Lipton RB, Dodick DW, Freitag FG, Ramadan N, Mathew N, et al. Efficacy and safety of topiramate for the treatment of chronic migraine: A randomized, double-blind, placebo-controlled trial. Headache. 2007;**47**(2):170-180

[143] Jackson JL, Cogbill E, Santana-Davila R, et al. A comparative effectiveness meta-analysis of drugs for the prophylaxis of migraine headache. PLoS One. 2015;**10**(7):e0130733

[144] Lainez MJ, Freitag FG, Pfeil J, et al. Time course of adverse events most commonly associated with topiramate for migraine prevention. European Journal of Neurology. 2007;**14**(8):900-906

[145] Silberstein SD, Goadsby PJ. Migraine: Preventive treatment. Cephalalgia. 2002;**22**:491-512

[146] Ruiz L, Ferrandi D. Topiramate in migraine progression. The Journal of Headache and Pain. 2009;**10**:419-422

[147] Limmroth V, Biondi D, Pfeil J, Schwalen S. Topiramate in patients with episodic migraine: Reducing the risk for chronic forms of headache. Headache. 2007;**47**:13-21

[148] Novartis Europharm Limited. Aimovig (erenumab) for Injection: Summary of Product Characteristics. 2018. Available from: https://www.ema.europa.eu/documents/product-information/aimovig-epar-product-information_en.pdf [Accessed: 11 July 2019]

[149] Amgen Inc. Aimovig™ (Erenumab-aooe) Injection, for Subcutaneous Use: US Prescribing Information

[150] Teva GmbH. Ajovy (Fremanezumab) for Injection: Summary of Product Characteristics. 2018. Available from: https://www.ema.europa.eu/documents/product-information/ajovy-epar-product-information_en.pdf [Accessed: 11 July 2019]

[151] Teva Pharmaceutical Industries Ltd. Ajovy™ (Fremanezumab-vfrm) Injection, for Subcutaneous Use. 2018. Available from: https://www.accessdata.fda.gov/drugsatfda_docs/label/2018/761089s000lbl.pdf [Accessed: 11 July 2019]

[152] Eli Lilly and Company. Emgality (Galcanezumab-glnm) Injection, for Subcutaneous Use: US Prescribing Information. 2018. Available from: https://www.accessdata.fda.gov/drugsatfda_docs/label/2018/761063s000lbl.pdf [Accessed: 11 July 2019]

[153] Eli Lilly Nederland BV. Emgality (Galcanezumab) for Injection: Summary of Product Characteristics. 2018. Available from: https://www.ema.europa.eu/en/documents/product-information/emgality-epar-product-information_en.pdf [Accessed: 11 July 2019]

[154] Lundbeck. Vyepti (Eptinezumab-jjmr): US Prescribing Information. 2020. Available from: https://www.lundbeck.com/upload/us/files/pdf/Products/Vyepti_PI_US_EN.pdf [Accessed: 05 March 2020]

[155] Dhillon S. Eptinezumab: First approval. Drugs. 2020;**80**:733-739

[156] Goldberg SW, Silberstein SD. Targeting CGRP: a new era for migraine treatment. CNS Drugs. 2015;**29**(6): 443-452

[157] Deen M, Correnti E, Kamm K, Kelderman T, Papetti L, Rubio-Beltran E, et al. Blocking CGRP in migraine patients - a review of pros and cons. The Journal of Headache and Pain. 2017;**18**(1):96

[158] Edvinsson L. CGRP receptor antagonists and antibodies against CGRP and its receptor in migraine treatment. British Journal of Clinical Pharmacology. 2015;**80**(2):193-199

[159] Israel H, Neeb L, Reuter U. CGRP monoclonal antibodies for the preventative treatment of migraine. Current Pain and Headache Reports. 2018;**22**(5):38

[160] Silberstein SD, Dodick DW, Bigal ME, Yeung PP, Goadsby PJ, Blankenbiller T, et al. Fremanezumab for the preventive treatment of chronic migraine. The New England Journal of Medicine. 2017;**377**:2113-2122

[161] Detke HC, Goadsby PJ, Wang S, Friedman DI, Selzler KJ, Aurora SK. Galcanezumab in chronic migraine: the randomized, double-blind, placebo-controlled REGAIN study. Neurology. 2018;**91**:e1-e11

[162] Dodic DW, Lipton RB, Silberstein S, et al. Eptinezumab for prevention of chronic migraine: A randomized phase 2b clinical trial. Cephalalgia. 2019;**39**(9):1075-1085

[163] Sacco S, Bendtsen L, Ashina M, et al. European headache federation

guideline on the use of monoclonal antibodies acting on the calcitonin gene related peptide or its receptor for migraine prevention. The Journal of Headache and Pain. 2019;**20**:6

[164] Tepper S, Ashina M, Reuter U, Brandes JL, Doležil D, Silberstein S, et al. Safety and efficacy of erenumab for preventive treatment of chronic migraine: a randomised, double-blind, placebo-controlled phase 2 trial. Lancet Neurology. 2017;**16**:425-434

[165] Bigal ME, Edvinsson L, Rapoport AM, Lipton RB, Spierings EL, Diener HC, et al. Silberstein SD (2015a) safety, tolerability, and efficacy of TEV-48125 for preventive treatment of chronic migraine: a multicentre, randomised, double-blind, placebo-controlled, phase 2b study. Lancet Neurology. 2015;**14**:1091-1100

[166] Yang M, Rendas-Baum R, Varon SF, et al. Validation of the Headache Impact Test (HIT-6) across episodic and chronic migraine. Cephalalgia. 2010;**31**:357-367

[167] Lipton RB, Goadsby PJ, Smith J, Schaeffler BA, Biondi DM, Hirman J, et al. Efficacy and safety of eptinezumab in patients with chronic migraine PROMISE-2. Neurology. 2020;**94**(13): e1365-e1377. DOI: 10.1212/WNL. 0000000000009169

[168] Kowacs F, Roesler CAP, Piovesan EJ, et al. Consensus of the Brazilian Headache Society on the treatment of chronic migraine. Arquivos de Neuro-Psiquiatria. July 2019:**77**(7): 509-520. DOI: 10.1590/0004-282x20190078

[169] Peroutka SJ. Beyond monotherapy: rational polytherapy in migraine. Headache. 1998;**38**(1):18-22

[170] Pellesi L, Do TP AH, et al. Dual therapy with anti-cgrp monoclonal antibodies and botulinum toxin for migraine prevention: Is there a rationale? Headache. 2020. DOI: 10.1111/head.13843

[171] Diener HC, Dodick DW, Goadsby PJ, et al. Chronic migraine—Classification, characteristics and treatment. Nature Reviews. Neurology. 2012;**32**:423

[172] Dodick DW. Finding a fit: Strategies for chronic migraine prophylaxis. Johns Hopkins Advanced Studies in Medicine. 2006;**6**(4D)

Chapter 6

Chronic Migraine in Adolescence

Marcos Antonio da Silva Cristovam, Daniel Albiero Piélak, Júlia Deitos, Júlia Natsumi Hashimoto, Lorena Vaz Meleiro Lopes and Luísa Manfredin Vila

Abstract

Chronic migraine (CM) is a clinically and epidemiologically important disease that generates considerable impairment to those affected by it, since there is evidence of higher incidence of depression, anxiety, and chronic pain in patients with this condition. It is characterized by the occurrence of headache for at least 8 migraine days in a month and at least 15 headache days in the same month. Despite the similarity in CM presented in adults, when in adolescents it has some particularities. Thus, the aim of this chapter was to conduct a literature review, using the databases: PubMed, SciELO, and LILACS, in addition to text books, explaining the definition, epidemiology, risk factors, diagnosis, pathophysiology, treatment, and prevention of CM in adolescent population.

Keywords: classic migraine, migraine with auras, epidemiology, adolescence, diagnosis

1. Introduction

Chronic migraine (CM) is defined as the occurrence of headache for at least 8 migraine days in a month and at least 15 headache days in the same month [1], being much less common and more debilitating than episodic migraine. Evidence indicates that migraine is a progressive disorder [2–4], and therefore, diagnosis and early management of episodic migraine are recommended, in order to avoid its chronicity, especially in adolescents; however, there is a failure in the accuracy of the diagnosis of CM in this population [5]. Migraine in this population can be misdiagnosed as sinusitis, attempted school skipping, and cerebral neoplasia, which may culminate in unnecessary testing [6].

2. Epidemiology

CM is a common disorder in children, and its incidence in adolescents presents a considerable increase [7]. Irrespective of age, the prevalence of chronic migraine is estimated at 1.5–2% in general population. On the other hand, its prevalence is 3% (from 3 to 7 years of age), 4–11% (from 7 to 11 years of age), and 8–23% (at 11 years of age), with a mean age of onset of 7.2 years for male and 10.9 years for female [8, 9]. Migraine is the 6th most disabling disease worldwide between the ages of 10 and 14 years and the 5th between the ages of 15 and 19 years [10]. In addition to toe the line impact inflicted by pain itself, migraine generates serious consequences in children's and adolescent's routine, since it is responsible for school absences, negatively affecting academic performance. It also has social impacts, since it hinders the child's interactions with his peers, and economic, due to the costs generated by the treatment [11]. Migraine has two-fold higher prevalence in females when compared to their peer male adolescents [12–17]. In women, the prevalence of migraine increases during adolescence, presenting a maximum prevalence at 30 years of age, decreasing sharply after menopause [12, 14, 17], since 50–60% of women report having migraine during their menstrual period [18]. In the American Migraine Prevalence and Prevention Study (AMPP), patients with CM presented with depression, anxiety, and chronic pain twice as much as patients with episodic migraine [17]. Abu-Arafeh et al., in 2010, estimated that the overall prevalence of migraine in children is 7.7% (9.7% in female and 6.0% in male), being more common in female after completing 11 years of age, in male before the age of 7, and being equal in both sexes between 7 and 11 years of age [19, 20]. In another study, WöberBingöl et al. reported general prevalence of migraine of 9.1% [21].

3. Risk factors

Among the risk factors for CM, the following are included:

a. gender (female, once migraine has been associated with menorrhagia, dysmenorrhoea, and endometriosis [22]);

b. age group;

c. ethnicity: more specifically, white;

d. genetic factors: family history of headache, mental disorders [5, 22, 23], anxiety, and depression [5, 23], as well as comorbidities, such as sleep disorders [5, 23] (sleep apnea syndrome and hypopnea, snoring, and insomnia [22]), obesity [23], epilepsy [24], hypertension, asthma, hypothyroidism, genitourinary disorders, musculoskeletal disorders, [22] and gastrointestinal disorders [22, 24];

e. family and environmental factors: divorce [23], socioeconomic class [5, 23], and low level of education [5]; and

f. other factors: pro-thrombotic factors [5] and pro-inflammatory factors [5, 23].

In addition to the factors mentioned above, others still under study may be related to the pathophysiology of CM and, therefore, represent risk factors such as traumatic brain injury, epilepsy, hemodialysis, and excessive use of symptomatic medications.

The existence of correlation between CM and traumatic brain injury was the subject of a systematic review study published by Sowell et al., in 2017, in which was sought to relate it to posttraumatic chronic headache (PTCH) in children and adolescents. In this study, it was observed that 7.6% of children with PTCH presented migraine [24], thus disclosing it to be a relatively common condition and that it should be considered.

Another factor that may be correlated with CM is epilepsy. Both migraine and epilepsy are considered neuronal hyperarousal-related diseases which can be partially prevented by antiepileptic drugs. According to the Center of Disease Control (CDC), 16.2% of adults with no history of epilepsy have severe headache or migraine, while those with active epilepsy have 35.5% of prevalence [25]. Therefore, although the correlation between epilepsy and migraine has not been completely elucidated yet, there are strong indications for such an interdependence.

Regarding hemodialysis in pediatric and adolescent patients with chronic kidney disease, Davidovits and Eidlitz Markus, in a study published in the International Headache Society, concluded a three-fold higher prevalence of headache among patients in hemodialysis compared to those with chronic kidney disease without this treatment, the most commonly described type of headache being migraine. Furthermore, other variables were associated with headaches, such as anemia, hyperparathyroidism, and low glomerular filtration [26].

Notwithstanding, excessive symptomatic medication is also described in the literature as a risk factor for CM. With this in mind, Rojo et al. made a comparison between patients with CM with and without excessive medication use (analgesics, tryptans, ergotamine, and opioids). In the study, it was observed that individuals overusing symptomatic medication had the onset of migraine at a younger age, with a longer progression time before looking for a specialist, as well as a higher percentage of preventive prior treatment (mainly antidepressants), compared to those without excessive use of medication [5].

4. Diagnosis

Even though there are differences between the clinical findings of CM in the pediatric population and other age groups, due to the scarce evidence in relation to diagnostic methods aimed specifically at these patients, the International Classification of Headache Disorders, of Headache Classification Committee of the International Headache Society (IHS), 2018, is used, the same applied to the adult population [1, 5].

According to IHS, CM is characterized by occurrence of ≥8 days of migraine in a month and ≥15 headache days. Migraine attacks can be with and/or without aura [1]. In this case, migraine without aura is a headache lasting 4–72 h, which has at least two of the following characteristics: (1) unilateral location; (2) pulsatile character; (3) moderate to strong pain intensity; and (4) is exacerbated by routine physical activities and, during the headache, the patient has at least one of the following symptoms: (1) nausea and/or vomiting; (2) photophobia; and (3) phonophobia [1].

On the other hand, migraine with aura is a headache with the same characteristics mentioned above, plus one or more symptoms of fully reversible aura, and may be visual, sensory, speech and/or language, motor, brain stem, or retinal. Furthermore, crises should have at least three of the following characteristics: (1) at least one symptom of aura gradually spreads for more than 5 min; (2) two or more aura symptoms occur in succession; (3) each individual aura symptom lasts 5–60 min; (4) at least one symptom of aura is unilateral; (5) at least one symptom of aura is positive; and (6) aura is accompanied, or followed within 60 min, by headache [1].

Although the use of IHS criteria is recommended, the health professional should know the peculiarities of CM in adolescent population in order to complement the diagnosis. The characteristics of the headache tend to be more prominent in this group, since the brain is in the growth and development process. Furthermore, the duration of pain crises may be less than 1 h, contrary to the IHS criteria, which mentions a minimum duration of 2 h [1, 6, 27]. A direct relation between the patient's age and duration of crises is observed, being younger shorter the duration of the crisis [4]. An important information is that adolescents may present nonpulsatile and bilateral pain, which may induce the misdiagnosis of tensional headache [2, 6, 27].

Approximately 10% of young people with migraine present aura, from visual, sensory, speech, or language disorders, motor, or brain stem changes, manifesting themselves as scotomas, paresthesias, dysphasias, hemiplegia, ataxia, or confusion. The suspicion of other diseases of the central nervous system should be listed through fever, nuchal stiffness, altered mental status, absence of family history of migraine, occipital or positional headaches, or headaches that constantly awaken the individual during sleep [28–30].

In adolescents, it is common for patients with migraine to have comorbidities such as epilepsy and atopy. The most common atopic disorders reported concomitantly with CM are seasonal rhinitis, conjunctivitis, and asthma, with correlation with positive family history. Regarding epilepsy, it is mainly associated with migraine with aura, which corroborates the role of depression of cortical propagation. Another hypothesis is that both, migraine and epilepsy, have the influence of canalopathies on their pathophysiology [30–32].

5. Pathophysiology

The mechanisms responsible for the occurrence of CM are not yet fully understood. Thus, the existing model to explain its pathophysiology still has gaps. It is accepted that migraine occurs by complex mechanisms involving activation and sensitization of trigeminal nociceptive pathways, especially its ophythalmic division, changes of the autonomic nervous system function, descending pain modulator system dysfunction, thalamic sensitization, and central sensitization due to the excessive use of medication in the acute treatment of pain crises.

It is noteworthy that the córtex of patients with migraine is hyperexcitable and abnormally sensitive to external stimuli. Due to triggering factors, the so-called cortical spreading depression (CSD) occurs, characterized by a slow propagation wave (2–6 mm/min) of sustained neuronal depolarization, which generates a transient peak of intense activity as it progresses in the tissue, followed by a long-term neural suppression. That is, there is a period of electrochemical hyperactivity followed by cortical inactivity, which results in the release of substances in the extracelular environment (ECE), such as K^+ and H^+ ions, nitric oxide, arachidonic acid, and prostaglandins [33–35]. Such a change in the ECE may activate or sensitize trigeminal afferences. The trigeminal ganglia, once stimulated, releases neuropeptides, causing inflammation of the dura mater. Cernuda-Morollón et al. demonstrate in their studies that interictal levels of calcitonin gene-related peptide (CGRP) and intestinal vasoactive peptide (IVP) are higher in CM [36, 37]. Thus, meningeal inflammation occurs, with vasodilation and endotelial dysfunction, resulting in plasma leakage and release of more inflammatory cytokines by mast cells. Thereby, neurogenic inflammation can lead to activation and sensitization of meningeal trigeminal afferences—a phenomenon known as peripheral sensitization [38–40].

A widely spread hypothesis is that increased peripheral nociceptive processing triggers increased activity of the descending pain modulation system, resulting in increased oxidative stress and consequent nociceptive modulation, further lowering the threshold for new pain crises. However, so far studies have not shown association between gene polymorphisms associated with oxidative stress and the occurrence of CM. On the other hand, repetitive painful stimuli on the trigeminal nerve cause activation of the pain modulating descending system in several portions, including the periaqueductal gray matter, showing that during migraine attacks, the neurons of this region show increased activity, which may lead to oxidative stress and finally dysfunction of nociceptive modulation by such system [33, 41–43].

Thalamic modulation of trigeminal afferences appears to be related to the development of cutaneous allodynia in migraine, as sensitized thalamic neurons process nociceptive information from cranial meninges, along with sensory information from the scalp, skin, face, body, and limbs. Furthermore, the use of drugs that act modulating trigeminal afferences on the thalamus is effective in the preventive treatment of migraine attacks, such as topiramate, sodium valproate, and CGR66 receptor antagonists, corroborating the role of this structure in the chronicity of migraine [44–47].

The overuse of medications to relieve acute migraine may also lead to the chronicity of this condition, through the drug-mediated central sensitization mechanism, leading to increased susceptibility to cortical spreading depression. Central sensitization manifests clinically from increased pericranial sensitivity and allodynia [48–50].

Andersen et al. demonstrated in 2016 that during pain crises serum miRNA changes occur, and in patients with CM such changes persist the same in periods without pain. This implies the possibility of serum miRNA changes as a pathogenic feature of migraine. Thus, the study suggests that serum miRNA dosage is a potential biomarker of this disease [51].

According to Oakley et al., there is a possibility that obesity may be involved in the pathophysiology of migraine in the pediatric population. It is hypothesized that there is an overlap of the central and peripheral neural pathways responsible for the regulation of diet and those linked to the pathogenesis of migraine [33, 52]. Peterlin et al. demonstrated that several hypothalamic peptides, proteins, and neurotransmitters involved in the mechanisms of hunger also participate in the pathophysiology of migraine, such as serotonin, orexin, and adipokines. It is possible that the release of these substances, associated with the mechanism of diet and/or obesity states, may act as a trigger or corroborate the development of migraine. There is also the possibility that lifestyle and behavioral differences influence the relationship between migraine and obesity, such as differences in diet and physical exercise, or the lack of it [33, 53].

6. Treatment

6.1 General and supportive measures

The treatment of chronic migraine in adolescents aims not only to reduce frequency, duration, and intensity of the headache attacks, but also to reduce the consequences of this condition on the patient's quality of life, seeing as he or she is going through a process of growth and development. It also aims to treat comorbidities and reduce the social impact of the disease, such as school absences, school underachievement, and reduced peer interactions. Thus, the treatment should be developed from a multiprofessional perspective, with the help of pediatricians, neurologists and psychiatrists, psychologists, educators, and nutritionists, among others [54].

Firstly, family members should receive detailed information about the adolescent's diagnosis and ensure that the condition is not secondary to malignant diseases, in order to transmit confidence to the patient and their parents, thus contributing to treatment adherence [5].

Proper living habits are of paramount importance for treatment. However, the health professional should be careful to not excessively restrict the activities of young people, as this may lead to difficulties in adherence [55].

Sleep disorders are important comorbidities of chronic migraine. Therefore, regular sleep habits should be advocated in order to promote restful and restorative sleep. For this, the teenager can use some techniques, such as scheduling a daily bedtime, avoid using electronic media when in bed, avoid eating 4 h before bedtime, and avoid daytime naps. Still, sleep deprivation can be a triggering factor for pain crises, corroborating the importance of a well-slept night [56, 57].

Regarding food, it is important to prioritize regular meals, with the consumption of healthy foods and adequate hydration. Caffeine and tobacco should be avoided. The performance of physical activities should be encouraged, as it not only reduces the occurrence of crises, but also is able to assist in the treatment of depression and anxiety comorbidities, when present [58, 59].

Gelfand et al. emphasize that the patient should be alerted about the negative effects of overuse of medications, as it is one of the factors responsible for the chronicity of migraine, from the central sensitization mechanism, as previously explained about the pathophysiology [60].

Kroon Van Diest et al. [61], based on a randomized study, demonstrated the importance of Cognitive Behavioral Therapy (CBT) for adherence to pharmacological treatment and institution of lifestyle changes [62]. CBT aims, through interventions guided by a psychologist, to promote the patient's active learning in order to implement skills to deal with migraine and related conditions and situations to her. Thus, during the sessions, behavioral coping skills are worked out, such as problem-solving and thought restructuring, that is, the adolescent is urged to change their ideas, beliefs, and attitudes regarding his chronic condition [62]. CBT, in combination with amitriptyline, is suggested as a first-line treatment in the context of CM in adolescents [61].

6.2 Acute treatment

Regarding acute pharmacological treatment, that is, to relieve pain crises, nonsteroidal anti-inflammatory drugs (NSAIDs) and triptans are used [28, 63, 64]. Among NSAIDs, the most used are ibuprofen and naproxen [28]. Evers et al. demonstrated that ibuprofen is better than placebo. There is no evidence regarding the efficacy of acetaminophen in adolescents [63, 65, 66].

In the adolescent population, the following triptans are indicated: sumatriptan, rizatriptan, zolmitriptan, and almotriptan. Studies indicate that such drugs are the most effective in relieving pain during acute crises in adolescents, with no statistically significant differences between them [63]. According to Derosier et al., the combination of naproxen and sumatriptan was superior to placebo when analyzing the permanence of analgesia after 2 h, with sumatriptan + naproxen sodium 10 mg + 60 mg (29%; $p = 0{,}003$), 30 mg + 180 mg (27%; $p = 0.003$), and 85 mg + 500 mg (24%; $p = 0.003$) versus placebo (10%) [67]. Among the side effects of this class, the most common are mild fatigue, paresthesia, dizziness, and taste disorders [28, 64].

In the case of long-term migraine or migratory status, that is, disabling crisis lasting more than 72 h, hospital treatment may be required for intravenous administration of prochlorperazine with ketorolac, which Brousseau showed that 57% of patients had pain reduction in 60 min [28, 68]. Dihydroergotamine (DHE) has been shown to be well tolerated and effective in acute treatment and is generally administered in hospital setting, and an association with metoclopramide or prochlorperazine is suggested, which is able to attenuate gastrointestinal side effects [28, 69]. Ayulo et al. suggested the use of intravenous lidocaine for the treatment of migratory status in adolescents, but further evidence is needed to ensure the long-term efficacy and safety of this medication [28, 70].

6.3 Preventive treatment

Prevention of chronic migraine attacks in adolescents remains limited [71, 72]. Newly developed therapies, including drugs, biologic products, and neuromodulation devices are safe and well tolerated in adults [73–80]. Studies in the pediatric population are still being developed [81]. Therefore, the current nonpediatric prevention will be presented.

Epidemiological studies suggest that approximately 38% of migraine patients require preventive therapy, however, only 3–13% currently use it [12]. The prevention of CM currently presents concrete evidence for the following drugs: onabotulinumtoxina [82], topiramate [83, 84], and fremanezumab (TEV-48125) [85]. Other therapies, such as β-blockers and amitriptyline, are often used despite the lack of evidence, as they are not fully effective or poorly tolerated, which may culminate in low adherence rates [85]. However, a randomized study developed by Powers et at. demonstrated that amitriptyline, when combined with Cognitive Behavioral Therapy (CBT), reduces migraine disability and pain days by 1 month—adolescents receiving amitriptyline alone (group A) reduced the number of days with headache in 1 month of 6.8 days, while those who associated amitriptyline with CBT (group B) had a reduction of 11.5 days; headache disability as assessed by the Pediatric Migraine Disability Score (PedMIDAS) decreased by 52.7 points in group B versus 38.6 points in group A [62].

Currently, new forms of prevention have been proposed, based on the understanding of the pathophysiology of the disease. The calcitonin gene-related peptide (CGRP) has increased plasma concentration during a migraine attack [86–88]. Therefore, a human monoclonal antibody against the receptor of CGRP, named Galcanezumab, which was effective in preventing migraine when given at a dose of 150 mg twice a month, was developed in a study by Skljarevski et al. [89]. Treatment with self-administered injections of subcutaneous galcanezumab [90], subcutaneous fremanezumab [91], and enerumab [92] was associated with a reduction in the number of monthly days of migraine (5.6–6.5 days, 1.3–1.5 days, and 6.6 days, respectively).

Recent studies indicate that nonpharmacological strategies are effective in preventing CM, reducing the activation of peripheral nociceptive terminations. This can be accomplished by manipulation technique, increasing the range of motion and reducing the stiffness of the cervicothoracic spine. In the study by Gandolfi et al., patients undergoing this treatment had lower consumption of analgesics, NSAIDs, and triptans [93].

Guilbot et al. showed that *Tanacetum parthenium* L., magnesium, and coenzyme Q10, administered prophylactically for 3 months significantly reduced the number of monthly migraine days (4.9 ± 2.6 days) [94]. Silberstein et al. proposed the prevention of CM with noninvasive vagal stimulation, which presented better results in patients who underwent longer treatment times (6 months, in the study) [95].

7. Conclusion

CM in adolescents is a disease of clinical and epidemiological importance, since it can affect approximately a quarter of the pediatric population with an average of 11 years of age, being considered debilitating due to psychological, social, and economic repercussions.

This disorder has intrinsic and nonmodifiable (genetic and comorbidities) risk factors, as well as modifiable risk factors, such as behavioral and socioenvironmental variables, in addition to several other elements still under study that may contribute to the onset or that are correlated.

The diagnosis of migraine is made clinically according to the ICHD-3 criteria, taking into account the particularities of the adolescent population.

Pathophysiology, as well as risk factors and prevention, are still not completely elucidated items in CM. However, it is generally agreed that migraine occurs from complex mechanisms involving activation and sensitization of trigeminal nociceptives pathways, alteration of autonomic nervous system function, pain modulating descending system dysfunction, thalamic sensitization and further central sensitization due to the overuse of medicines in the acute treatment of pain crises.

Treatment, in turn, is multiprofessional and supported by both pharmacological and nonpharmacological measures. Nonpharmacological measures include guidance to parents and family members about the chronic condition, as well as sleep hygiene and adoption of good eating habits by the patient. In the case of drug measures, NSAIDs and triptans are the first option and, in case of migraine status, prochlorperazine associated with intravenous ketorolac added to recent evidence suggesting the use of intravenous lidocaine.

Finally, studies are still needed to fill the gaps present for the complete understanding of this complex and debilitating entity that is chronic migraine. Through a better understanding of the pathophysiological mechanisms responsible for the development of CM, as well as its risk factors, it will be possible to develop more effective prevention and treatment methods in adolescents.

Author details

Marcos Antonio da Silva Cristovam[1*], Daniel Albiero Piélak[2], Júlia Deitos[3], Júlia Natsumi Hashimoto[3], Lorena Vaz Meleiro Lopes[3] and Luísa Manfredin Vila[3]

1 Clinical Pediatrics of Western Paraná State University, Cascavel, PR, Brazil

2 Western Paraná Universitary Hospital of Western Paraná State University, Cascavel, PR, Brazil

3 Western Paraná State University School of Medicine, Cascavel, PR, Brazil

*Address all correspondence to: ma.cristovam@uol.com.br

References

[1] Headache Classification Committee of the International Headache Society (IHS). The international classification of headache disorders. Cephalalgia. 2018;**38**(1):1-211

[2] Lipton RB, Silberstein SD. Episodic and chronic migraine headache: Breaking down barriers to optimal treatment and prevention. Headache. 2015;**55**(2):103-122

[3] Lipton RB, Pan J. Is migraine a progressive brain disease? Journal of the American Medical Association. 2004;**291**(4):493-494

[4] Lipton RB, Bigal ME. Migraine: Epidemiology, impact, and risk factors for progression. Headache. 2005;**45**(1):3-13

[5] Özge A, Yalın OÖ. Chronic migraine in children and adolescents. Current Pain and Headache Reports. 2016;**20**(2):1-7. DOI: 10.1007/s11916-016-0538-z

[6] Gelfand AA. Migraine in young children. Developmental Medicine and Child Neurology. 2015;**57**(6):503

[7] Victor TW, Hu X, Campbell JC, Buse DC, Lipton RB. Migraine prevalence by age and sex in the United States: A life-span study. Cephalalgia. 2010;**30**:1065-1072

[8] Stewart WF, Linet MS, Celentano DD, Van Natta M, Siegler D. Age and sex-specific incidence rates of migraine with and without visual aura. American Journal of Epidemiology. 1991;**34**:1111-1120

[9] Stewart WF, Lipton RB, Celentano DD, Reed ML. Prevalence of migraine headache in the United States. Journal of the American Medical Association. 1992;**267**:64-69

[10] GBD 2015 Disease and Injury Incidence and Prevalence Collaborators. Global, regional, and national incidence, prevalence, and years lived with disability for 310 diseases and injuries, 1990-2015: A systematic analysis for the Global Burden of Disease Study 2015. Lancet. 2016;**388**:1545-1602

[11] Arruda MA, Bigal ME. Migraine and migraine subtypes in preadolescent children: Association with school performance. Neurology. 2012;**79**:1881-1888

[12] Lipton RB, Bigal ME, Diamond M, Freitag F, Reed ML, Stewart WF. Migraine prevalence, disease burden, and the need for preventive therapy. Neurology. 2007;**68**:343-349

[13] Bigal ME, Liberman JN, Lipton RB. Age-dependent prevalence and clinical features of migraine. Neurology. 2006;**67**:246-251

[14] Steiner TJ, Scher AI, Stewart WF, Kolodner K, Liberman J, Lipton RB. The prevalence and disability burden of adult migraine in England and their relationships to age, gender and ethnicity. Cephalalgia. 2003; **23**:519-527

[15] Ando N, Fujimoto S, Ishikawa T, et al. Prevalence and features of migraine in Japanese junior high school students aged 12-15 yr. Brain & Development. 2007;**29**:482-485

[16] Zencir M, Ergin H, Sahiner T, et al. Epidemiology and symptomatology of migraine among school children: Denizli urban area in Turkey. Headache. 2004;**44**:780-785

[17] Lipton RB, Stewart WF, Diamond S, Diamond ML, Reed M. Prevalence and burden of migraine in the United States: Data from the American migraine study II. Headache. 2001;**41**:646-657

[18] Granella F, Sances G, Zanferrari C, Costa A, Martignoni E, Manzoni GC. Migraine without aura and reproductive life events: A clinical epidemiological study in 1300 women. Headache. 1993;**33**:385-389

[19] Abu-Arafeh I, Razak S, Sivaraman B, et al. Prevalence of headache and migraine in children and adolescents: A systematic review of population-based studies. Developmental Medicine and Child Neurology. 2010;**52**(12):1088-1097

[20] Mehta S. Study of various social and demographic variables associated with primary headache disorders in 500 school-going children of central India. Journal of Pediatric Neurosciences. 2015;**10**(1):13

[21] Wöber-Bingöl Ç. Epidemiology of migraine and headache in children and adolescents. Current Pain and Headache Reports. 2013;**17**(6):1-11

[22] Spierings ELH, Padamsee A. Menstrual-cycle and menstruation disorders in episodic vs chronic migraine: An exploratory study. Pain Medicine. 2015;**16**(7):1426-1432. DOI: 10.1111/pme.12788

[23] Rojo E, Pedraza MI, Muñoz I, Mulero P, Ruiz M, de la Cruz C, et al. Diferencias entre migraña crónica con y sin uso excesivo de medicación: Experiencia en una serie hospitalaria de 434 pacientes. Neurología. 2015;**30**(3):153-157. DOI: 10.1016/j.nrl.2013.12.003

[24] Sowell MK, Youssef PE. The comorbidity of migraine and epilepsy in children and adolescents. Seminars in Pediatric Neurology. 2016;**23**(1):8391. DOI: 10.1016/j.spen.2016.01.012

[25] Shaw L, Morozova M, Abu-Arafeh I. Chronic post-traumatic headache in children and adolescents: Systematic review of prevalence and headache features. Pain Management. 2018;**8**(1):57-64. DOI: 10.2217/pmt-2017-0019

[26] Davidovits M, Eidlitz Markus T. Headache in pediatric and adolescent patients with chronic kidney disease, with and without hemodialysis: A comparative cohort study. Cephalalgia. 2017;**38**(5):883-891. DOI: 10.1177/0333102417719235

[27] Mariani R, Torriero R, Capuano A, et al. Clinical characteristics of primary headaches in children younger than 6 years. Cephalalgia. 2015;**35**:7-7

[28] Slater SK, Powers SW, O'Brien HL. Migraine in children. Current Opinion in Pediatrics. 2018;**1**:775-778. DOI:10.1097/mop.0000000000000694

[29] Lewis DW, Ashwal S, Dahl G, et al. Practice parameter: Evaluation of children and adolescents with recurrent headaches: Report of the quality standards Subcommittee of the American Academy of neurology and the practice Committee of the Child Neurology Society. Neurology. 2002;**59**:490-498

[30] Newton RW. Childhood headache. Archives of Disease in Childhood. Education and Practice Edition. 2008;**93**:105

[31] Özge A, Öksüz N, Ayta S, et al. Atopic disorders are more common in childhood migraine and correlated headache phenotype. Pediatrics International. 2014;**56**(6):868-872

[32] Bellini B, Arruda M, Cescut A, et al. Headache and comorbidity in children and adolescents. The Journal of Headache and Pain. 2013;**14**(1):79

[33] May A, Schulte LH. Chronic migraine: Risk factors, mechanisms and treatment. Nature Reviews Neurology. 2016;**12**(8):455-464. DOI: 10.1038/nrneurol.2016.93

[34] Durham P, Papapetropoulos S. Biomarkers associated with migraine and their potential role in migraine management. Headache: The Journal of Head and Face Pain. 2013;**53**(8): 1262-1277. DOI: 10.1111/head.12174

[35] Vecchia D, Pietrobon D. Migraine: A disorder of brain excitatory-inhibitory balance? Trends in Neurosciences. 2012;**35**:507-520

[36] Cernuda-Morollón E et al. Increased VIP levels in peripheral blood outside migraine attacks as a potential biomarker of cranial parasympathetic activation in chronic migraine. Cephalalgia. 2015;**35**:310-316

[37] Cernuda-Morollón E et al. Interictal increase of CGRP levels in peripheral blood as a biomarker for chronic migraine. Neurology. 2013;**81**:1191-1196

[38] Waeber C, Moskowitz MA. Migraine as an inflammatory disorder. Neurology. 2005;**64**:S9-S15

[39] Levy D. Migraine pain, meningeal inflammation, and mast cells. Current Pain and Headache Reports. 2009;**13**:237-240

[40] Pietrobon D, Moskowitz MA. Pathophysiology of migraine. Annual Review of Physiology. 2013;**75**(1): 365-391. DOI: 10.1146/annurev-physiol-030212-183717

[41] Schulte LH, Sprenger C, May A. Physiological brainstem mechanisms of trigeminal nociception: An fMRI study at 3T. NeuroImage. 2015;**124**:518-525

[42] Youssef AM, Macefield VG, Henderson LA. Pain inhibits pain; human brainstem mechanisms. NeuroImage. 2016;**124**(Pt A):54-62

[43] Gentile G et al. Lack of association between oxidative stress-related gene polymorphisms and chronic migraine in an Italian population. Expert Review of Neurotherapeutics. 2015;**15**:215-225

[44] Burstein R et al. Thalamic sensitization transforms localized pain into widespread allodynia. Annals of Neurology. 2010;**68**:81-91

[45] Andreou AP, Goadsby PJ. Topiramate in the treatment of migraine: A kainate (glutamate) receptor antagonist within the trigeminothalamic pathway. Cephalalgia. 2011;**31**:1343-1358

[46] Andreou AP, Shields KG, Goadsby PJ. GABA and valproate modulate trigeminovascular nociceptive transmission in the thalamus. Neurobiology of Disease. 2010;**37**:314-323

[47] Summ O, Charbit AR, Andreou AP, Goadsby PJ. Modulation of nocioceptive transmission with calcitonin gene-related peptide receptor antagonists in the thalamus. Brain. 2010;**133**(9):2540-2548. DOI: 10.1093/brain/awq224

[48] De Felice M et al. Triptan-induced latent sensitization: A possible basis for medication overuse headache. Annals of Neurology. 2010;**67**:325-337

[49] Green AL et al. Increased susceptibility to cortical spreading depression in an animal model of medication-overuse headache. Cephalalgia. 2014;**34**:594-604

[50] Becerra L et al. Triptans disrupt brain networks and promote stress-induced CSD-like responses in cortical and subcortical areas. Journal of Neurophysiology. 2016;**115**:208-217

[51] Andersen HH, Duroux M, Gazerani P. Serum MicroRNA signatures in Migraineurs during attacks and in pain-free periods. Molecular Neurobiology. 2015;**53**(3):1494-1500. DOI: 10.1007/s12035-015-9106-5

[52] Oakley CB, Scher AI, Recober A, Peterlin BL. Headache and obesity in the pediatric population. Current Pain and Headache Reports. 2014;**18**(5):1-12. DOI: 10.1007/s11916-014-0416-5

[53] Peterlin BL, Tietjen GE, Gower BA, et al. Ictal adiponectin levels in episodic migraineurs: A randomized pilot trial. Headache. 2013;**53**:474-490

[54] De Angelis V, Cherubini F, Nigrelli G, Erbuto D, Marteletti P. Multimodal therapy in the management of MOH: 3 year experience. The Journal of Headache and Pain. 2015;**16**:135

[55] Sieberg CB, Huguet A, von Baeyer CL, Seshia S. Psychological interventions for headache in children and adolescents. The Canadian Journal of Neurological Sciences. 2012;**39**(01):26-34

[56] Guidetti V, Dosi C, Bruni O. The relationship between sleep and headache in children: Implications for treatment. Cephalalgia. 2014;**34**(10):767-776

[57] Calhoun AH, Ford S. Behavioral sleep modification may revert transformed migraine to episodic migraine. Headache. 2007;**478**(11):787-811

[58] Straube A, Heinen F, Ebinger F, von Kries R. Headache in school children: Prevalence and risk factors. Deutsches Ärzteblatt International. 2013;**6**(57):811-818

[59] Verotti A, Di Fonzo A, Penta L, Agostinelli S, Parisi P. Obesity and headache/migraine: The importance of weight reduction through lifestyle modifications. BioMed Research International. 2014;**2014**:420858

[60] Gelfand AA, Goadsby PJ. Medication overuse in children and adolescents. Current Pain and Headache Reports. 2014;**18**(7):1-6

[61] Kroon Van Diest AM, Ramsey RR, Kashikar-Zuck S, Slater S, Hommel K, Kroner JW, et al. Treatment adherence in child and adolescent chronic migraine patients. The Clinical Journal of Pain. 2017;**33**(10):892-898. DOI: 10.1097/ajp.0000000000000481

[62] Powers SW, Kashikar-Zuck SM, Allen JR, et al. Cognitive behavioral therapy plus amitriptyline for chronic migraine in children and adolescents: A randomized clinical trial. Journal of the American Medical Association. 2013;**310**(24):2622-2630

[63] Richer L, Billinghurst L, Linsdell MA, Russell K, Vandermeer B, Crumley ET, et al. Drugs for the acute treatment of migraine in children and adolescents. Paediatrics & Child Health. 2017;**22**(8):454-458. DOI: 10.1093/pch/pxx170

[64] Patniyot IR, Gelfand AA. Acute treatment therapies for pediatric migraine: A qualitative systematic review. Headache. 2016;**56**:49-70

[65] Evers S, Rahmann A, Kraemer C, Kurlemann G, Debus O, Husstedt IW, et al. Treatment of childhood migraine attacks with oral zolmitriptan and ibuprofen. Neurology. 2006;**67**(3):497-499. DOI: 10.1212/01.wnl.0000231138.18629.d5

[66] Lewis DW, Kellstein D, Dahl G, Burke B, Frank LM, Toor S, et al. Children's ibuprofen suspension for the acute treatment of pediatric migraine. Headache. 2002;**42**(8):780-786. DOI: 10.1046/j.1526-4610.2002.02180.x

[67] Derosier FJ, Lewis D, Hershey AD, Winner PK, Pearlman E, Rothner AD, et al. Randomized trial of sumatriptan and naproxen sodium combination in adolescent migraine. Pediatrics. 2012;**129**(6):e1411-e1420. DOI: 10.1542/peds.2011-2455

[68] Brousseau DC, Duffy SJ, Anderson AC, Linakis JG. Treatment of pediatric migraine headaches: A randomized, double-blind trial of prochlorperizine versus ketorolac. Annals of Emergency Medicine. 2004;**42**:256-262

[69] Kabbouche MA, Powers SW, Hershey AD, et al. Inpatient treatment of status migraine with dihydroergotamine in children and adolescents. Headache. 2009;**49**:106-109

[70] Ayulo MA Jr, Philips KE, Tripathi S. Safety and efficacy of IV Lidocaine in the treatment of children and adolescents with status migraine. Pediatric Critical Care Medicine. 2018;**19**:755-759

[71] Lewis D, Ashwal S, Hershey A, et al. Practice parameter: Pharmacological treatment of migraine headache in children and adolescents: Report of the American Academy of Neurology quality standards subcommittee and the practice Committee of the Child Neurology Society. Neurology. 2004;**63**:2215-2224

[72] Jackson JL. Pediatric migraine headache—Still searching for effective treatments. The New England Journal of Medicine. 2017;**376**:169-170

[73] Silberstein SD et al. Fremanezumab for the preventive treatment of chronic migraine. The New England Journal of Medicine. 2017;**377**:2113-2122

[74] Misra UK, Kalita J, Bhoi SK. High frequency repetitive transcranial magnetic stimulation (rTMS) is effective in migraine prophylaxis: An open labeled study. Neurological Research. 2012;**34**:547-551

[75] Goadsby PJ, Reuter U, Hallström Y, et al. A controlled trial of erenumab for episodic migraine. The New England Journal of Medicine. 2017;**377**:2123-2132

[76] Detke HC, Goadsby PJ, Wang S, Friedman DI, Selzler KJ, Aurora SK. Galcanezumab in chronic migraine: 10 month 2019 the randomized, double-blind, placebo-controlled REGAIN study. Neurology. 2018;**91**:e2211-e2221

[77] Chou DE, Shnayderman Yugrakh M, Winegarner D, Rowe V, Kuruvilla D, Schoenen J. Acute migraine therapy with external trigeminal neurostimulation (ACME): A randomized controlled trial. Cephalalgia. 2019;**39**:3-14

[78] Martelletti P, Barbanti P, Grazzi L, et al. Consistent effects of non-invasive vagus nerve stimulation (nVNS) for the acute treatment of migraine: Additional findings from the randomized, sham-controlled, double-blind PRESTO trial. The Journal of Headache and Pain. 2018;**19**:101

[79] Kuca B, Silberstein SD, Wietecha L, et al. Lasmiditan is an effective acute treatment for migraine: A phase 3 randomized study. Neurology. 2018;**91**:e2222-e2232

[80] Voss T, Lipton RB, Dodick DW, et al. A phase IIb randomized, double-blind, placebo-controlled trial of ubrogepant for the acute treatment of migraine. Cephalalgia. 2016;**36**:887-898

[81] Hornik CP, Gelfand AA, Szperka CL, Pezzuto T, Utevsky A, Kessel S, et al. Development of a prospective real-world data clinical registry of children and adolescents with migraine. Headache: The Journal of Head and Face Pain. 2019;**0**:2-9. DOI: 10.1111/head.13714

[82] Dodick DW, Turkel CC, DeGryse RE, et al. OnabotulinumtoxinA for treatment of chronic migraine: Pooled results from the double-blind, randomized, placebo-controlled phases of the PREEMPT clinical program. Headache. 2010;**50**:921-936

[83] Silberstein S, Lipton R, Dodick D, et al. Topiramate treatment of chronic migraine: A randomized, placebo-controlled trial of quality of life and other efficacy measures. Headache. 2009;**49**:1153-1162

[84] Silberstein SD, Lipton RB, Dodick DW, et al. Efficacy and safety of topiramate for the treatment of chronic migraine: A randomized, double-blind, placebo-controlled trial. Headache. 2007;**47**:170-180

[85] Bigal ME, Edvinsson L, Rapoport AM, et al. Safety, tolerability, and efficacy of TEV-48125 for preventive treatment of chronic migraine: A multicentre, randomised, double-blind, placebo-controlled, phase 2b study. Lancet Neurology. 2015;**14**:1091-1100

[86] Goadsby PJ, Edvinsson L, Ekman R. Vasoactive peptide release in the extracerebral circulation of humans during migraine headache. Annals of Neurology. 1990;**28**(2):183-187

[87] Goadsby PJ, Edvinsson L. The trigeminovascular system and migraine: Studies characterizing cerebrovascular and neuropeptide changes seen in humans and cats. Annals of Neurology. 1993;**33**(1):48-56

[88] Juhasz G, Zsombok T, Modos EA, et al. NO-induced migraine attack: Strong increase in plasma calcitonin gene-related peptide (CGRP) concentration and negative correlation with platelet serotonin release. Pain. 2003;**106**(3):461-470

[89] Skljarevski V, Oakes TM, Zhang Q, Ferguson MB, Martinez J, Camporeale A, et al. Effect of different doses of galcanezumab vs placebo for episodic migraine prevention. JAMA Neurology. 2018;**75**(2):187. DOI: 10.1001/jamaneurol.2017.3859

[90] Camporeale A, Kudrow D, Sides R Wang S, Van Dycke A, Selzler KJ, et al A phase 3, long-term, open-label safet study of Galcanezumab in patients wit migraine. BMC Neurology. 2018;**18**(1): 1-10. DOI: 10.1186/s12883-018-1193-2

[91] Dodick DW, Silberstein SD, Bigal ME, Yeung PP, Goadsby PJ, Blankenbiller T, et al. Effect of Fremanezumab compared with placebo for prevention of episodic migraine. Journal of the American Medical Association. 2018;**319**(19):1999. DOI: 10.1001/jama.2018.4853

[92] Tepper S, Ashina M, Reuter U, Brandes JL, Doležil D, Silberstein S, et al. Safety and efficacy of erenumab for preventive treatment of chronic migraine: A randomised, double-blind, placebo-controlled phase 2 trial. The Lancet Neurology. 2017;**16**(6):425-434. DOI: 10.1016/s1474-4422(17)30083-2

[93] Gandolfi M, Marchioretto F, Turrina A, Dimitrova E, Geroin C, Valè N. Does myofascial and trigger point treatment reduce pain and analgesic intake in patients undergoing OnabotulinumtoxinA injection due to chronic intractable migraine? A pilot, single-blind randomized controlled trial. European Journal of Physical and Rehabilitation Medicine. 2017;**54**(1):1-12

[94] Guilbot A, Bangratz M, Ait Abdellah S, Lucas C. A combination of coenzyme Q10, feverfew and magnesium for migraine prophylaxis: A prospective observational study. BMC Complementary and Alternative Medicine. 2017;**17**(1):1-6. DOI: 10.1186/s12906-017-1933-7

[95] Silberstein SD, Calhoun AH, Lipton RB, Grosberg BM, Cady RK, Dorlas S, et al. Chronic migraine headache prevention with noninvasive vagus nerve stimulation. Neurology. 2016;**87**(5):529-538. DOI: 10.1212/wnl.0000000000002918

Section 4

The New Headache Problem on the Scene

Chapter 7

Medication Overuse Headache

Dhruv Bansal, Pritesh Pranay and Fayyaz Ahmed

Abstract

Medication overuse headache (MOH) is defined in the latest ICHD-3 criteria as a secondary headache caused by worsening of a pre-existing headache (usually a primary headache) owing to overuse of one or more attack-aborting or pain-relieving medications. MOH can be debilitating and results from biochemical and functional brain changes induced by certain medications taken too frequently. Various risk factors some modifiable, other non-modifiable (Multiple Gene Polymorphisms) have been hypothesised in MOH. Psychiatric co-morbidities in MOH are noticeably (anxiety and depression) found to be co morbid disorders by more than chance. This has to be managed effectively along with treatment strategies for MOH for efficacious response to withdrawal treatment. Ample literature and clinical evidence shown in prospective trials, that withdrawal therapy is the best treatment for MOH. The mainstay of MOH treatment is not only to detoxify the patients and to stop the chronic headache but also, most likely, to improve responsiveness to acute or prophylactic drugs. Studies advocating prophylactic treatment with good response to mainly topiramate and OnabotulinumtoxinA do exist, less prominent for prednisolone, however, not recommended for every patient. Management may be complex and must be done via MDT approach with involvement of specialists when needed along with incorporating adequate treatment of acute withdrawal symptoms, educational and behavioural programs to ensure patient understanding of the condition and compliance. There are arguments on either sides of inpatient and outpatient withdrawal for MOH patients dependent heavily on the individual circumstances i.e. patient's motivation, the duration of the overuse, the type of overused drugs, possible previous history of detoxification failures and co morbidities. Treatment trials are still required to determine for clinicians the best evidence-based approach for helping these patients break their headache cycle.

Keywords: medication overuse, chronic migraine, chronic daily headaches, rebound headaches, painkillers

1. Introduction

Medication-overuse headache (MOH) is defined by the International Classification of Headache Disorders (ICHD) as a headache in patients with primary headache disorders occurring on ≥15 days per month for >3 months, that is induced by overuse of medications taken as symptomatic treatment for acute headaches.

In ICHD-3, chronic headache syndromes are described by professional consensus as headache disorders that share traits with pre-existing headache syndromes, happen for a specific duration of time (at least three months in Chronic tension-type headache (CTTH), Chronic migraine (CM); or at least 12 months in Chronic trigeminal autonomic cephalalgia (TAC)) and have an extra time-rule (e.g.headache days per month in CTTH and CM, or the absence of remissions for greater than three months in TAC's).

MOH occurs if the number of days of acute medicine taken for headache per month exceeds a threshold level [1] i.e., 15 or more days for simple painkillers and 10 or more days for triptans, opioids and combination analgesics. The diagnosis of MOH as per ICHD-3 is given as follows:

2. Diagnosis of medication-overuse headache

2.1 According to the ICHD-3 beta diagnostic criteria1, each of the criteria A–C have to be fulfilled for the diagnosis of medication overuse headache

A

- Headache on ≥15 days/month
- Pre-existing headache disorder

B

- Overuse of acute and/or symptomatic headache medications for >3 months*C
- Not better represented by any other ICHD-3 diagnosis

*Regular consumption of tablets on ≥10 days/month for ergotamines, triptans, opioids and mixture analgesics and on ≥15 days/month for paracetamol (also recognised as acetaminophen), acetylsalicylic acid and NSAIDs.

As ICHD defines MOH as a secondary headache, one must identify the primary headache disorder associated with it for example episodic or chronic migraine. The classification identifies further sub-groups based on the substance misused (e.g., 2.2.1.2 triptan-overuse headache). Many sufferers take more than one drug [2] or are overusing combination analgesics and/or multiple drugs at different times which are identified in the classification as headache attributed to numerous drug classes (2.2.5). The comprehensive classification of MOH from ICHD-3 is given here:

2.2 International classification of headache disorders third edition (ICHD-3) criteria for medication-overuse headache (MOH)

2.2.1 Medication-overuse headache (MOH)

A. Headache happening on ≥15 days/month in a affected person with a pre-existing headache disorder

B. Regular overuse for > three months of one or more drugs that can be taken for acute and/or symptomatic treatment of headache

C. Not better represented by means of any other ICHD-3 diagnosis.

2.2.1.1 Ergotamine-overuse headache

A. Headache satisfying standards for 2.2.1 Medication- overuse headache

B. Regular consumption of ergotamine on ≥10 days/month for >three months.

2.2.1.2 Triptan-overuse headache

A. Headache satisfying criteria for 2.2.1 Medication- overuse headache

B. Regular consumption of one or greater triptans, 1 in any formulation, on ≥10 days/month for >3 months.

2.2.1.3 Non-opioid analgesic-overuse headache

2.2.1.3.1 Paracetamol (acetaminophen)-overuse headache

A. Headache satisfying criteria for 2.2.1 Medication- overuse headache

B. Regular consumption of paracetamol on ≥15 days/month for > three months.

2.2.1.4 Non-steroidal anti-inflammatory drug (NSAID)- overuse headache

A. Headache satisfying criteria for 2.2.1 Medication- overuse headache

B. Regular consumption of one or extra non-steroidal anti- inflammatory drugs (NSAIDs) (other than acetylsalicylic acid) on ≥15 days/month for >3 months.

2.2.1.4.1 Acetylsalicylic acid-overuse headache

A. Headache satisfying criteria for 2.2.1 Medication- overuse headache

B. Regular intake of acetylsalicylic acid on ≥15 days/month for >three months.

2.2.1.5 Other non-opioid analgesic-overuse headache

A. Headache satisfying criteria for 2.2.1 Medication- overuse headache

B. Regular intake of a non-opioid analgesic other than paracetamol or non-steroidal anti-inflammatory tablets (including acetylsalicylic acid) on ≥15 days/month for> three months.

2.2.2 Opioid-overuse headache

A. Headache satisfying criteria for 2.2.1 Medication- overuse headache

B. Regular consumption of one or more opioids on ≥10 days/month for >3 months.

2.2.3 Combination-analgesic-overuse headache

A. Headache fulfilling standards for 2.2.1 Medication- overuse headache

B. Regular consumption of one or more combination-analgesic medicines on ≥10 days/month for >three months.

2.2.4 Medication-overuse headache attributed to combination drug classes not individually overused

A. Headache satisfying standards for 2.2.1 Medication- overuse headache

B. Regular intake of any aggregate of ergotamine, triptans, non-opioid analgesics and/or opioids on a total of ≥10 days/month for >3 months besides overuse of any single drug or drug type alone.

2.2.5 Medication-overuse headache attributed to unspecified or unverified overuse of numerous drug classes

A. Headache satisfying standards for 2.2.1 Medication- overuse headache

B. Both of the following: 1. regular consumption of any mixture of ergotamine, triptans, non-opioid analgesics and/or opioids on ≥10 days/month for >3 months

2.2.6 Medication-overuse headache attributed to different medication

A. Headache fulfilling standards for 2.2.1 Medication- overuse headache

B. Regular overuse, on ≥10 days/month for >3 months, of one or greater medicines other than these described above, 1 taken for acute or symptomatic cure of headache

3. Background and pathophysiology

MOH was first identified in 1951 in relation to overuse of ergotamine [3]. It was in 1984 that relationship between analgesic consumption and exacerbation of headaches were recognised with improvement in headaches on stopping them [4]. It was given the name as 'drug-induced headache' in the first classification of the headache disorders (ICHD-1) [5]. The ICHD-2 described this as 'medication-overuse headache' in 2004. The condition was said to be probable as the definitive diagnosis was only given following reduction of headache days 2 months after withdrawal of the overused medication [6]. The 2006 modification broadened the definition [7] by abolishing the required improvement after discontinuation and this has persisted in both ICHD-3 beta and ICHD-3 criteria [8].

4. Clinical characteristics

The headache of medication overuse is that of the primary headache disorder [9]. Patients with migraines who overuse triptan will observe increase in the frequency of pre-existing headaches to almost daily in frequency that exacerbates intermittently and more so if a dose of triptan is missed. The patient gets in a vicious circle with increasing headaches proportional to the triptans consumed. In the same way patients with tension-type headache will report exacerbation of their featureless headaches [9]. A few people are able to differentiate between their primary headaches and a constant dull and diffuse headache that they attribute as MOH. It has been observed that MOH develops more quickly with triptan and resolves more quickly on withdrawal compared to combination and simple analgesics. This perception was confirmed by a French study [10].

The diagnostic criteria for MOH do not fully demonstrate the complexity of making the diagnosis of MOH. It is important to realise that medication overuse and MOH are two different entities that can have different implications and outcomes. Medication-overuse only signifies the number of days a person consumes painkiller and not necessarily a cause for on-going headache. In certain chronic painful conditions e.g., back pain; arthritis etc. there is medication overuse but no accompanying headache. Another observation has been that not every individual will develop headache with acute medication overuse [11]. It is not entirely clear why overuse worsens headache in some and not the others. Considered a secondary headache disorder, MOH should be identified by the type of medication being overused. The primary headache disorder must also be identified.

5. Prevalence and general risk factors

Majority of research have reported the general prevalence of MOH in the normal population to be 0.5–2.6% [12]. Higher rates have been seen in Russia (7.6%) [13] and Iran (4.6%), where medication overuse is a lot more frequent than in other nations [14]. However, no speculative reason or hypothesis has been provided for this.

The prevalence for MOH is 0.5–2.6% although it varies based on the availability of painkillers over the counter (OTC) and hence reported much higher in Russia (7.6%) and Iran (4.6%). The availability of OTC varies with codeine-based analgesics available in the UK, while barbiturates containing painkillers in the USA. Figures from the third world countries such as India and Pakistan are difficult to obtain considering all forms of painkillers are available over the counter with no definitive prescription system existing in the country. The prevalence is less common in adolescents (0.3%–0.5%) than adults observed in two epidemiological studies in Norway and Taiwan [15, 16]. Overall females are affected more than males (5:4) and those with chronic migraine have a very high incidence of medication overuse (11–70%) much more than observed in the general population [17].

6. Risk factors

On the basis of current scientific knowledge, all pain medications have the capacity to cause MOH. Dependency-like behaviour is most commonly seen in patients who overuse opioids, although it is also seen in patients overusing triptans [18–20]. Medication overuse was found to be an important risk factor for chronification of primary headaches [21]. A study in the USA found majority of patients with medication overuse were taking combined painkillers containing caffeine or opioids than simple painkillers [22]. They concluded that the risk of MOH is less with simple painkillers although this does not prove a link between overuse and a specific medication.

In a large prospective population-based study, Hagen et al. studied 25.596 patients who did not suffer from chronic daily headache at baseline but had MOH 11 years later (n = 201,0.8%) and the risk factors that were found to be associated with development of MOH: regular use of tranquillisers, combination of chronic musculoskeletal complaints, gastrointestinal complaints and hospital anxiety depression scale (HADS) score > =11, physical inactivity and smoking [23]. Migraine headaches was more strongly linked with MOH than non-migraine headaches and the risk was higher with those having a high frequency i.e., 7–14 days per month, although it remains unclear as to whether this is because of a higher analgesic intake or frequent migraine attacks. Some of the non-modifiable risk factors for MOH include young age, female gender, family history of analgesic or substance overuse and low education level. Smoking and physical inactivity were other risk factors for MOH that were not associated with chronic daily headache without medication overuse suggesting that the two conditions are phenotypically different [23]. In 80% of patients with MOH, migraine is the underlying primary headache disorder [24] and majority of remaining patients have tension-type headache or more rarely post traumatic headache [25–27].

7. Main risk factors for MOH

RISK FACTOR OR (95% CI)
Demographics
AGE(<50 years) 1.8(1.3–2.4)
Female sex 1.9(1.4–2.6)
Low degree of education 1.9(1.2–3.0)
Complaints that were self-disclosed
Chronic Musculoskeletal problems 1.9(1.4–2.7)
Gastrointestinal problems 1.6(1.1–2.2)
Depression or Anxiety (HADS score ≥ 11) 4.7(2.4–9.0)
Medications
Tranquillisers 5.2(3.0–9.0)
Aspirin 0.5(0.3–0.9)
Ibuprofen 0.7(0.5–1.0)
Opioids 2.3(1.3–3.9)
Lifestyle
Smoking 1.8(1.2–2.5)
Physical Inactivity 2.7(1.2–6.3)
Metabolic Syndrome 5.3(1.6–24.6)
High daily Caffeine intake 1.4(0.8–2.5) (>540 mg versus ≤240 mg)

Figure shown are derived from population-based studies [23] in Norway [15, 16], the USA [22] and China.CI, confidence interval; HADS, Hospital Anxiety and Depression; MOH, medication-overuse headache; OR, odds ratio.

8. Pathophysiology

The pathophysiology of MOH remains unclear. The fact that patients with migraine or tension type headache are more likely to develop MOH may mean that the underlying mechanism for MOH could be related to a brain with these primary headache disorders [28]. Patients with cluster headache (another primary headache disorder) do not develop MOH in spite of regular painkillers unless they also suffer from or have a family history for migraine [29]. It is possible that a genetic risk

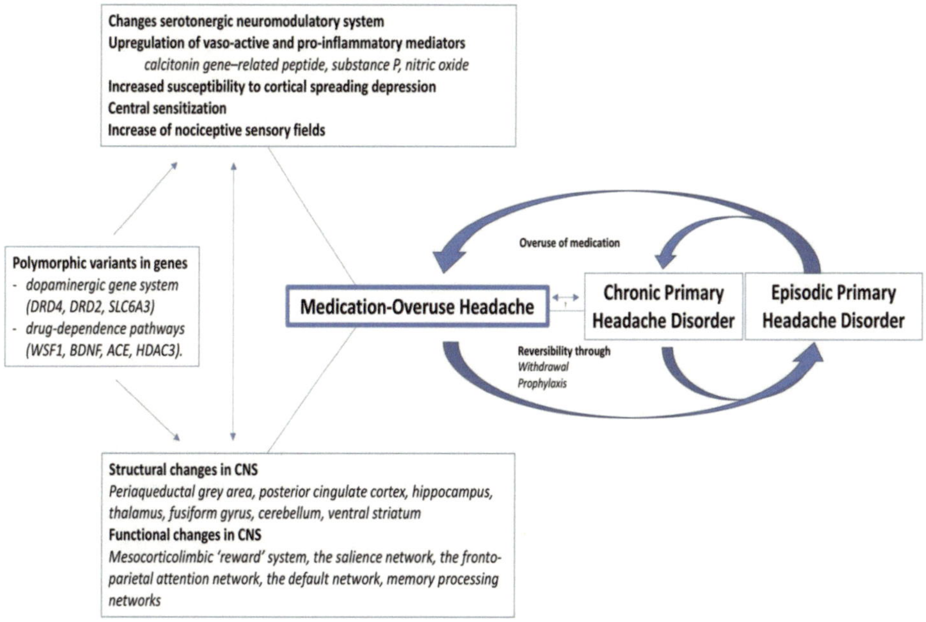

Figure 1.
Current perception of the pathophysiology of medication-overuse headache (MOH) [30]. The understanding on the pathophysiology of MOH entails transformation from and reversion to primary headache disorders, displaying changes in physiological processes, functional connectivity, and structural changes of the central nervous system, in patients with underlying genetic predisposition. Abbreviations: MOH: Medication-overuse headache; CNS: Central nervous system (figure obtained from article 'medication overuse headache: A widely recognised entity amidst on-going debate' (open access)) [30] (http://creativecommons.org/licenses/by/4.0/).

factor in a migrainous brain could make the person more susceptible to MOH (**Figure 1**).

9. Genetic risk factors

9.1 Angiotensin-converting enzyme polymorphism

The renin-angiotensin system is well known for blood pressure control. Angiotensin II can cause increase in blood pressure and require Angiotensin-converting enzyme (ACE) for its formation from Angiotensin I. It also has a role in regulating neural plasticity [31] and its interaction with monoaminergic synaptic transmission contributes towards dependence behaviour [32]. Polymorphism (insertion/deletion) in the gene that encodes ACE may well play a role in the condition particularly the D/D genotype [33].

9.2 Brain derived neurotrophic factor polymorphism

Brain-derived neurotrophic factor (BDNF) has been linked to substance overuse [34, 35]. Certain BDNF genotypes (non G/G) [36, 37] are associated with increased consumption behaviour for the painkillers than others.

9.3 Serotonin transporter polymorphism

Many affective disorders such as depression, anxiety and substance abuse are associated with variants of SLC6A4 that encodes for SERT (Serotonin transporter) [38, 39].

Patients with SLC6A4 variants that have MOH are extremely difficult to respond to withdrawal therapy and have a high relapse rate following withdrawal [40].

9.4 Catechol-O-methyltransferase (COMT) polymorphism

COMT is an enzyme that metabolises catecholamines such as dopamine, adrenaline and nor-adrenaline and influences pain modulation [41]. Certain genotypes of COMTSNP (rs4680 and rs6269) have a low rate of relapse following withdrawal of analgesics than others indicating its role [40].

10. Pain medications role

All forms of painkillers are associated with MOH although certain classes of analgesics can cause the condition much quicker than others. For example patients with triptan overuse develop MOH much quicker than opioids, ergotamine and combination analgesics [42]. In the same way triptans withdrawal responds much quicker and has a much lower relapse rate. This indicates that the underlying pathophysiological mechanism may be medication specific. Platelets of those with migraine and medication overuse have higher 5-HT2 receptors than those without medication overuse [43]. The research has also shown a reduction of serotonin levels and a reduction of the primary endogenous cannabinoids, anandamide and 2-acylglycerol in those with Migraine and medication overuse compared to those without it [44]. Research has also shown that those with MOH have a high consumption of other medicines such as nasal decongestants, eye drops, laxatives, tranquillisers and sleeping drugs.

11. Activation of trigeminovascular system

One of the pathways for head pain in migraine is activation of the trigeminal primary afferent neurons innervating the intracranial and dural blood vessels. Stimulation of these vessels have shown to induce pain similar to migrainous headache [45, 46], although the exact underlying mechanism that activates the trigeminovascular system remains unclear. Among possible explanations include the spreading depression with subsequent neuronal depolarisation and activation of the trigeminovascular system and release of chemicals that produce neurogenic inflammation around the intracranial and dural blood vessels. Chronic use of paracetamol has shown to be associated with an increased activation of the nociceptive pathway involved in headache. Hence it is proposed that prolonged exposure to analgesics may lead to MOH via up-regulation of neural regulators of vasodilation and neurogenic inflammation. It has been known for some time that sustained systemic delivery of morphine exposure increases CGRP content in dorsal root ganglion neurons [47, 48]. Plentiful studies documenting continuous, persistent exposure of rats to triptans for a period of days was shown to result in a marked increase in the numbers of trigeminal ganglion cell bodies expressing CGRP and a modest increase in expression of substance P.

Imaging studies have demonstrated functional [49–51], structural [52, 53] and metabolic [54] adjustments of the central pain network in patients with MOH. In a voxel-based morphometric study [55] of individuals with MOH, grey matter volume was increased in the thalamus, midbrain, and striatum, and reduced in the frontal regions [52] that resolved in sufferers who show clinical improvement of

MOH [53]. Another study indicated that grey matter volume of the orbitofrontal cortex estimated response to medication-overuse treatment [56].

Functional MRI studies have shown MOH associated hypoactivitiy in certain cortical region including the right supramarginal gyrus, right inferior and superior parietal area that constitute the lateral pain system [49, 50]. This was further demonstrated in PET study where hypometabolism was also demonstrated in thalami and cerebellar vermis [54]. These changes resolved at the end of the overuse except in the orbito-frontal cortex [54]. It is to be emphasised that such changes are not unique to MOH and can be seen to some extent in other headache disorders (migraine) and pain conditions [55].

12. CO-morbidities

Co- morbidity is defined as the presence of one and more additional conditions co-occurring with a primary condition. Psychiatric co-morbidities in MOH are noticeably frequent and have been studied extensively since the earliest literature of patients with MOH [57]. MOH and mood disorders such as anxiety and depression are thought to be co morbid disorders by more than chance [57–60].

In the Norwegian BIMOH study, (double-blind pragmatic cluster randomised controlled trial carried out among 50 general practitioners in Norway) sixty MOH patients and 40 population controls were included. The MOH patients had significantly higher headache disability and anxiety scores than the population controls. Hospital Anxiety and Depression Scale (HADS) scores were collected in patients with MOH (before and after a brief intervention) and controls. MOH patients were found to show significantly higher HADS scores for anxiety [61].

In the European and Latina "COMOESTAS" trial, (694 patients with MOH from six centres had been included, of whom 492 completed the study) in a seven-month cohort study. The study used Hospital Anxiety and Depression (HAD) scoring and found more than half (56%) of MOH patients had anxiety while 40% suffered from depression [62]. Similar findings were seen in the 'Eurolight' trial conducted in ten European countries. The association was considerably stronger in contrast to a group of patients with migraine without overuse [63]. A study on Sodium Valproate in Medication Overuse Headache (SAMOHA) found substantially higher number of patients with moderate to severe anxiety compared to those with episodic migraine or healthy controls [64]. Moreover, MOH are more likely to have one or more psychiatric co-morbidities and some authors found a third of patient with clinically relevant obsessive–compulsive disorders (OCD) [65].

Subclinical OCD may be an additional risk factor for chronic headaches [64, 65]. MOH can also be associated to substance-related disorder spectrum, moreover since MOH and dependence share common neurobiological pathways; noticeably MOH patients do not share common personality characteristics seen with drug addicts [66, 67].

In a Chinese cohort, an association was found between MOH and metabolic disturbances namely obesity and hypertension was shown in female patients [68]. A Danish cross-sectional analysis confirmed an association between MOH and those metabolic derangements (smoking, physical inactivity and obesity, although causality could not be proven [69]. Lastly, patients with chronic headache and MOH present with a high prevalence of sleep symptomatology [70].

13. Treatment

There is adequate evidence that withdrawal therapy is the best treatment for MOH. The aim is not only to break the cycle of regular analgesic consumption but to improve responsiveness to both acute and prophylactic medications [71]. The following questions remain under discussion among headache experts:

1. Should preventive treatments be commenced at the time or following withdrawal of the analgesics?

2. Should the withdrawal be abrupt or gradual?

3. Should this be done as out-patient or done through in-patient admission.

13.1 Preventive treatment before or following withdrawal

There is argument on both sides and researchers are divided with respect to whether prophylactic medications are given at the time of withdrawal or after withdrawal. Study conducted in Germany found all patients should be offered a non-drug treatment and in the majority, additional preventive drug therapy. Taking evidence from randomised controlled trials into consideration, topiramate or OnabotulinumtoxinA should be offered as a treatment for this condition. About 50% of patients with chronic migraine and medication overuse will respond and show a significant reduction in headache days [72]. Similar results were seen with OnabotulinumtoxinA treatment in a large prospective study from Hull, UK. OnabotulinumtoxinA significantly reduced the headache and migraine days whilst increasing headache-free days and the benefit is equally seen in those with or without co-existing medication overuse. We acknowledge the value of analgesic withdrawal although we recommend that this can be achieved alongside preventive treatment [73].

No study has ever compared abrupt withdrawal with tapered withdrawal in prospective randomised trials; therefore, no formal evidence-based recommendation or guideline can be deduced. However, the majority of headache specialists consider drug withdrawal to be more effective if done abruptly than gradual [74–76].

13.2 Abrupt or gradual withdrawal

Abrupt withdrawal is recommended for overuse of triptans, ergots, paracetamol, aspirin and NSAIDs and could be done in outpatients. Most patients have a less protracted suffering and resolution of withdrawal symptoms is much quicker. Those on opioids, barbiturates, benzodiazepines and combination analgesics a tapered withdrawal is more appropriate as withdrawal symptoms are more severe. Patients are warned that their headaches may get worse before getting better and symptoms of nausea, vomiting, sleep disturbances, palpitations, restlessness and anxiety are troublesome for a week to 10 days and in some cases may persist for up to 4 weeks before showing improvement. The duration of worsening is shorter with triptans (4.1 days) than ergotamine (6.7 days) and NSAID (9.5 days) [77].

A study in Italy of 137 patients aiming to study the effectiveness of an educational strategy (advice to withdraw the overused medication/s) with that of two structured pharmacological detoxification programmes in patients with complicated medication overuse headache (MOH) plus migraine concluded that inpatient withdrawal is significantly more effective than advice alone or an outpatient strategy in complicated MOH patients [78]. Another multicentre study (N = 376) on MOH subjects in four European and two Latin American centres comparing in-patient or out-patient detoxification programme with optional prophylaxis and a follow up for 6 months concluded equal effectiveness of both strategies with or without prophylaxis [79]. Carlsen et al. (N = 72) in a prospective, outpatient study randomised patients to two groups with one taking no analgesic or acute migraine-medication and the other restricted to no more than two days of painkillers per week. Patients were followed up for 12 months. The primary outcome was percentage reduction in headache days per month after 6 months. The outcome was better in complete withdrawal and more patients reverted to episodic migraine in this group [80].

13.3 Inpatient or outpatient

The decision has to be taken on individual circumstances that include the type of overused medication, length of the overuse, patients' motivation and history of previous detoxification failures and presence of co-morbidities. Out-patient withdrawal is more suited to simple analgesic, brief overuse period and highly motivated patients [81]. Evidence in favour of inpatient withdrawal comes from an observational study from Austria showing statistically significant improvement of quality of life, depression and anxiety at 6-month follow-up [82]. Alternatively a study conducted in Milan has shown that direct comparison between inpatient withdrawal and outpatient withdrawal treatment showed that both methods were effective and revealed a significant reduction in headache days per month after 12 months and a decrease in the scores of migraine disability without superiority of one method [83].

There is no standardised accepted protocol for both in-patient withdrawal. Every clinic use their own method that does include intravenous dehydration, complete stoppage of oral painkillers and treatment with anti-emetics and intramuscular painkillers as and when required with or without steroids [84–88].

With respect to corticosteroids, there is low evidence for change in various headache outcome measures (i.e. use of rescue medication, days with severe or moderate headache, days without headache, headache days, and frequency of headache) [89, 90]. There is plentiful literature evidence to suggest that majority of patients will get worse before they get better [91].

14. Prophylaxis

Early and effective prophylaxis remains the key to avoid chronification of episodic migraine. As nearly two-thirds of patients with chronic migraine have co-existing medication overuse, the question remains largely unanswered whether prophylaxis should commence before or after analgesic withdrawal. There are arguments on both sides and the jury remains out as to which approach is better. Some argue that patients with previous failure would show a good prophylactic response following withdrawal [92]; others recommend prophylaxis at the same time as withdrawal [93].

There are open-label studies showing improved outcome for using valproic acid and topiramate in patients with chronic daily headache with medication overuse. A double-blind study on topiramate in patients with chronic migraine and medication overuse showed reduction of migraine days per month significantly higher in the topiramate group (−3.5 vs. 0.2 in placebo $p < 0.05$), although side effects were considerably higher in the topiramate group (75% versus 37% in placebo) [94]. This supported using topiramate use before analgesic withdrawal although the reduction on headache days were not large enough to change it to episodic form. A similar observation was observed in another topiramate study where the reduction in migraine days per month was significantly higher for topiramate than placebo (6.4 versus 4.7) [95].

In a Danish study consisting of 335 patients with MOH where abrupt detoxification was initiated, the headache frequency was reduced by 67% in migraine patients and by 37% in those with combined migraine and tension-type headache after a 2-month observation period without prophylactic medication [92]. There are randomised controlled trials to show that with patients affected by chronic migraine and MOH suggest the use of onabotulinumtoxinA and topiramate without early discontinuation. However, the quality of the data is limited due to the fact that it is based on post hoc analysis [96]. Two further studies in the states have shown improvement in headache days in patients with chronic migraine and medication overuse treated with onabotulinumtoxinA and concluded that withdrawal prior to prophylaxis may not be required in all patients with MOH [97].

15. Bridging therapy

Steroids and NSAID have so far been studied but their effectiveness remains inconclusive. Few studies have used a short course of steroids as bridging treatment with different outcomes. The first study from Brazil used a short course of oral prednisolone in an out-patient setting. They studied 400 patients with daily headaches for longer than 6 months. Symptomatic medications were stopped suddenly and prednisone was initiated in tapering doses during 6 days, followed by the introduction of preventive treatment. The study found eighty-five per cent of the patients experienced a reduction in headache frequency and no patients presented severe attacks during the first 6 days. 10 day follow up, 46% of the patients experienced at least 2 days without headache and 58% less intense attacks [98]. Another German randomised, placebo-controlled, double-blind study showed efficacy of prednisone for the treatment of withdrawal symptoms in patients with MOH (N = 20). The total number of hours with severe or moderate headache within the first 72 and 120 h was significantly lower in the prednisone group. The results show that prednisone might be effective in the treatment of medication withdrawal headache [99]. Another randomised, double-blind, and placebo controlled Norwegian study negated the use of steroids as prophylaxis in MOH. Patients (N = 100) were randomly assigned to prednisolone or placebo pills for six days. Study concluded prednisolone has no effect on withdrawal headache in unselected patients with chronic daily headache and medication overuse [100]. A brief period of prophylaxis with naproxen 500 mg bd for 10–20 days has been recommended based on experience [101], there are other doses used for different durations [102, 103].

16. Prognosis of withdrawal treatment

As a rule of thumb, overuse of acute treatment can lead to a poor prognosis of chronic headache and lower quality of life by itself [104]. The outcome for MOH patients withdrawing from their acute treatments has been reported in multiple literature citations. An accepted endpoint as mentioned in many studies for good response to therapy is a ≥ 50% reduction from baseline headache frequency and/or headache index. Successful withdrawal was found in around 50–70% of MOH patients after 1 year [105–113]. Managing to retain full withdrawal after 1 year was found to be a good predictor for long-term success [114, 115].A successful withdrawal leads to a better response for prophylactic treatment, even in patients with little improvement in headache frequency [116].Tension-type headache have documented to have a higher relapse risk [105–107, 117, 118]. Patients who kept overusing medication in the long-term had a poor response to withdrawal therapy and had a higher frequency of chronic headache [114]. Risk factors for short term relapse (1 year) were: high number of acute treatments, smoking, alcohol consumption and return to overused drugs [119]. Patients withdrawn from triptans have a lower relapse risk, while combined drug therapy had a higher relapse rate [106, 118, 120]. Drugs with codeine, low self-reported sleep quality and high self-reported bodily pain are probable predictors for poor outcome after 1 yr. [113]. A prospective study from Germany followed 96 patients with MOH of which 75 completed 4 years. 26 patients (31%) relapsed within first six months and a total of 32 (41%) in the first year. The following three years only two more relapsed totalling 34 (45%). The authors concluded that most of the patients who relapse do that in the first year (94%) and the long-term success is dependent on the type of primary headache and the type of overused painkiller [121].

Most recent evidence on the most effective treatment strategy comes from an Open-label, randomised clinical trial to compare 3 treatment strategies for MOH [122] which was conducted at the Danish headache Centre, Glostrup form October 2016 to June 2019. Random assignments (1:1:1 allocation) to 1 of the 3 outpatient treatments consisted of [1] Withdrawal Plus Preventive treatment [2] Preventive treatment without Withdrawal, or [3] Withdrawal with optional Preventive treatment 2 months after Withdrawal. The Primary outcome was change in the headache days per month after 6 months. Of 120 patients, 102 completed the 6 month follow-up and the headache days per month were reduced by 12.3 (95% CI, 9.3–15.3) in the withdrawal plus preventive group, by 9.9 (95% CI,7.2–12.6) in the preventive group, and by 8.5 (95% CI 5.6–11.5) in the withdrawal group (P = 0.20). In the withdrawal plus preventive group, 23 of 31 patients (74.2%) reverted to episodic migraine, compared with 21 of 35 (60%) in the preventive group and 15 of 36 (41.7%) in the withdrawal group (P = 0.03). Moreover, 30 of 31 patients (96.8%) were cured of MOH in the withdrawal plus preventive group, compared with 26 of 35 (74.3%) in the preventive group and 32 of 36 (88.9%) in the withdrawal group (P = 0.03). These findings correspond to a 30% (RR, 1.3; 95% CI 1.1–.16) increased chance of MOH cure in the withdrawal plus preventive group compared with the preventive group (P = 0.03), therefore based on these findings, withdrawal therapy combined with preventive medication from the start of the withdrawal is recommended as the preferred management for MOH.

17. Conclusion

MOH is a common and worldwide problem with a prevalence of 1% in the general population but accounts for nearly 11 to 70% in those with chronic daily headaches, often under-recognised and un treated correlates with a significant negative impact on the patient's quality of life. Opiates and combination analgesics carry an increased risk for MOH needs to be recognised and accepted as per literature. Among the multiple risk factors for the development of MOH, some are noted to be modifiable and require MDT approach for attention and action. Anxiety and depression are the most common co morbidities, and up to approximately 50% of patients show dependence-type behaviours like tolerance or inability to control pain medication usage.

Treatment trials are still required to determine for clinicians the best evidence-based approach for helping these patients break their obnoxious headache cycle (?), but intervention will require patient counselling, detoxification, and prevention therapy. The future needs to be tailored to include a focus on increased awareness of

MOH for the general population and primary prevention strategies for patients and providers. To achieve success in treatment, it is essential that the primary care provider, nurse practitioner, pharmacist, and hospital doctors openly communicate with the neurologist when MOH is suspected.

Author details

Dhruv Bansal[1], Pritesh Pranay[1] and Fayyaz Ahmed[1,2]*

1 Hull University Teaching Hospitals NHS Trust, Hull Royal Infirmary, Anlaby Road Hull HU3 2JZ

2 Hull York Medical School

*Address all correspondence to: fayyaz.ahmed@hey.nhs.uk

References

[1] Headache Classification Committee of the International headache society. The international classification of headache disorders 3rd edition(beta version). *Cephalalgia* **33**,629-808(2013).

[2] Bigal, M., Rapoport, A., Sheftell, F., Tepper, S. & Lipton, R. Transformed migraine and medication overuse in a tertiary headache centre-clinical characteristics and treatment outcomes. *Cephalalgia* **24**, 483-490(2004).

[3] Peters, G.& Horton,B.Headache:with special reference to the excessive use of ergotamine preparations and withdrawl effects.*Proc.Staff Meet.Mayo Clin.* **26**, 153-161(1951).

[4] Dichigans,J. *et al*. Analgetika-induzieter Dauerkopfschmerz. *Dtsch. Med.Wochenschr*.109,369-373(in German) (1984).

[5] Diener,H.C.& Wilkinson,M.(eds) *Drug Induced Headache*(Springer,1088). (1988).

[6] Headache Classification SubCommittee of the International headache society. The international classification of headache disorders:2nd edition. *Cephalalgia* **24**, (Suppl.1),9-160 (2004).

[7] Olesen,J.*et al*. New appendix criteria open for a border concept of chronic migraine. *Cephalalgia* **26**,724-746 (2006).

[8] Headache Classification Committee of the International Headache Society (2018) Headache Classification Committee of the International Headache Society(IHS) the international Classification of headache disorders, 3rd Edition.

[9] Limmorth, V., Katsarava, Z., Fritsche, G., Przywara, S.& Diener,H. Features of medication overuse headache following overuse of different acute headache drugs. *Neurology* 59,1011-1014(2002).

[10] Creac'h, C.et al. One or several types of triptan overuse headache. *Headache* **49**, 519-528(2009).

[11] Martelletti P. The journey from genetic predisposition to medication overuse headache to its acquisition as sequela of chronic migraine. *J Headache Pain*. 2018;19(1):2.

[12] Westergaard M.L., Hansen, E.H., Glumer, C., Olesen, J.&Jensen, R.H. Definitions of medication overuse headache in population-based studies and their implications on prevalence estimates: a systematic review. *Cephalagia* **34**, 409-425 (2014).

[13] Ayzenberg, I.*et al*. The prevalence of primary headache disorders in Russia: a countyrwide survey. *Cephalalgia* **32**, 373-381(2012).

[14] Shahbeigi, S. *et al*. Epidemiology of headache in Tehran urban area: a population-based cross-sectional study in district 8, year 2010. *Neuol. Sci*. **34**, 1157-1166(2013).

[15] Dybs, G., Homen, T.L.&Zwart, J.A. Analgesic overuse among adolescents with headache: the Head-HUNT-Youth study. *Neurology* **66**, 198-201(2006).

[16] Wang, S.J., Fuh, J.L.,Lu,S.R.&Juang, K.D. Chronic daily headache in adolescents: prevalence, impact, and medication overuse. *Neurology* **66**, 193-197(2006).

[17] Westergaard M.L., Glumer, C., Hansen, E.H. & Jensen, R.H. Prevalence of chronic headache with and without medications overuse: associations with socioeconomic position and physical and mental health status. *Pain* 155, 2005-2013(2014).

[18] Radat, F.*et al*. Behavioral dependence in patients with medication overuse headache: a cross-sectional study in consulting patients using the DSM-IV criteria. *Headache* **48**, 1026-1036(2008).

[19] Lundqvist, C. Aaseth, K., Garnde, R. B., Benth, J.S.& Russell, M.B. The severity of dependence score correlates with medication overuse in persons with secondary chronic headaches. The Akershus study of chronic headache. *Pain* **148**, 487-491 (2010).

[20] Corbelli, I., Caproni, S., Eusebi, P.& Sarchiellli, P. Drug dependence behaviour and outcome of medictions overuse headache after treatment. *J. Headache Pain* **13**, 653-660(2012).

[21] Ashina S, Lyngberg A, Jensen RH (2010) Headache characteristics and chronification of migraine and tension-type headache: a population-based study. *Cephalalgia* **30**:943:954. https://doi.org/10.1177/03331024099357958

[22] Scher,A.I., Lipton, R.B.,Stewart, W. F.& Bigal, M.Patterns of medication use by chronic and episodic headache sufferers in the general population: results from the frequent headache epidemiology study. *Cephalalgia* **30**,321-328(2010).

[23] Hagen K, Albretsen C, Vilming ST *et al* (2001) A 4-year follow-up of patients with medication-overuse headache previously included in a randomised multicentre study. *J Headache Pain* **12**:315-322. http://doi.org/10.1007/s10194-010-0285-1

[24] Shand, B. *et al*. Clinical and demographical characteristics of patients with medication overuse headache in argentina and chile: analysis of latin American section of COMOESTAS project. *J.Headache Pain* 16, 83(2015).

[25] Hoem Nordhaug, L.etal. Headache in patinets with previous head injuries: a population-based historical cohort study (HUNT). Cephalalgia http://dx.doi.or/10.1177/0333102415618949 (2015)

[26] Heyer, G. L. & Idris, S. A. Does analgesic overuse contribute to post traumatic headaches in adolescent concussion patients? *Pediatr. Neurol.* **50**,464-468(2014).

[27] Knackstedt, H. et al. Cervicogenic headache in the general population: the Akershus study of chronic headache. *Cephalalgia* **30**, 1468-1476(2010).

[28] Lance,F.,parkes, C.& Wilkinson,M. Does analgesic abuse cause headaches de novo. *Headache* **28**, 61-62(1988).

[29] Paemeleire, K., Bahra, A., Evers,S., Matharu, M.S.&Goadsby, P.J. Medication-overuse headache in patients with cluster headache. *Neurology* **67**, 109-113(2006).

[30] Vandenbussche et al. Medication-overuse headache: a widely recognised entity amidst ongoing debate. *The Journal of headache and pain* (2018) 19: 50 http://doi.org10.1186/s10194-018-0875-x

[31] Phillips, M.I. Functions of angiotensin in the central nervous system. *Annu. Rev. Physiol*. **49**, 413-435 (1987).

[32] Pan, H.L. Brain angiotensin II and synaptic transmission. *Neuroscientist* **10**, 422-431(2004).

[33] Di Lorenzo, C.et al. Cortical response to somatosensory stimulation in medication overuse headache patients is influenced by angiotensin converting enzyme (ACE)I/D genetic polymorphism. *Cephalalgia* **32**, 1189-1197(2012).

[34] Binder,D.K.,&Scharfman, H.E. Barin-derived neurotrophic factor. *Growth Factors* **22**, 123–131 (2004).

[35] Gratacos, M. *et al.* Brain-derived neurotrophic factor Val66Met and psychiatric disorders: meta-analysis of case-control studies confirm association to substance-related disorders, eating disorders, and schizophrenia. *Biol. Psychiatry* **61**, 911–922 (2007).

[36] Bath, K. G. & Lee, F. S. Variant BDNF (Val66Met) impact on brain structure and function. *Cogn. Affect. Behav. Neurosci.* **6**, 79–85 (2006).

[37] DiLorenzo, C. *et al*. Drug consumption in medication overuse headache is influenced by brain-derived neurotrophic factor Val66Met polymorphism. *J. Headache Pain* **10**, 349–355 (2009).

[38] Serretti, A., Calati, R., Mandelli, L. & De Ronchi, D. Serotonin transporter gene variants and behavior: a comprehensive review. *Curr. Drug Targets.* **7**, 1659–1669 (2006).

[39] Kumar *et al.* Serotonin transported gene (SLC6A4) polymorphism in patients with irritable bowel syndrome and healthy controls. *J. Gastrointestin. Liver Dis.* **21**, 31–38 (2012).

[40] Cargnin, S. *et al.* Functional polymorphisms in COMT and SLC6A4 genes influence the prognosis of patients with medication overuse headache after withdrawal therapy. *Eur. J. Neurol.* **21**, 989–995 (2014).

[41] Andersen, S. & Skorpen, F. Variation in the *COMT* gene: implications for pain perception and pain treatment. *Pharmacogenomics* **10**, 669–684 (2009).

[42] DeFelice, M. *et al.* Triptan-induced latent sensitization: a possible basis for medication overuse headache. *Ann. Neurol.* **67**, 325–337 (2010).

[43] Srikiatkhachorn, A. & Anthony, M. Serotonin receptor adaptation in patients with analgesic-induced headache. *Cephalalgia* **16**, 419–422 (1996).

[44] Rossi, C., Pini, L. A., Cupini, M. L., Calabresi, P. & Sarchielli, P. Endocannabinoids in platelets of chronic migraine patients and medication-overuse headache patients: relation with serotonin levels. *Eur. J. Clin. Pharmacol.* **64**, 1–8 (2008).

[45] Ayata C.Spreading depression:from serendipity to targeted therapy in migraine prophylaxis.Cephalalgia 2009; 29:1095-1114.

[46] Ray BS and Wolff HG. Experimental studies on headache pain sensitive structures of the head and their significance in headache.Arch Surg 1940;41:813-856 .

[47] Belanger S, Ma W, Chabot JG, et al. Expression of Cal-citonin gene-related peptide, substance P and protein kinase C in cultured dorsal root ganglion neurons following chronic exposure to mu, delta and kappa opiates. *Neuroscience* 2002; 115: 441–453.

[48] Menard DP, van Rossum D, Kar S, et al. A calcitonin gene-related peptide receptor antagonist prevents the development of tolerance to spinal morphine analgesia. *J Neurosci* 1996; 16: 2342–2351.

[49] Grazzi, L. *et al.* Chronic migraine with medication overuse pre-post withdrawal of symptomatic medication: clinical results and FMRI correlations. *Headache* **50**, 998–1004 (2010).

[50] Ferraro, S. *et al.* Pain processing in medication overuse headache: a functional magnetic resonance imaging (fMRI) study. *Pain Med.* **13**, 255–262 (2012).

[51] Ferraro, S. *et al.* In medication-overuse headache, fMRI shows long-lasting dysfunction in midbrain areas. *Headache* **52**, 1520–1534 (2012).

[52] Riederer, F. *et al.* Grey matter changes associated with medication-overuse headache: correlations with disease related disability and anxiety. *World J. Biol. Psychiatry* **13**, 517–525 (2012).

[53] Riederer, F. *et al.* Decrease of gray matter volume in the midbrain is associated with treatment response in medication-overuse headache: possible influence of orbitofrontal cortex. *J. Neurosci.* **33**, 15343–15349 (2013).

[54] Fummal, A. *et al.* Orbitofrontal cortex involvement in chronic analgesic-overuse headache evolving from episodic migraine. *Brain* **129**, 543–550 (2006).

[55] Hu, W., Guo, J., Chen, N., Guo, J. & He, L. A meta- analysis of voxel-based morphometric studies on migraine. *Int. J. Clin. Exp. Med.* **8**, 4311–4319 (2015).

[56] Lai, T. H. *et al.* Gray matter changes related to medication overuse in patients with chronic migraine. *Cephalalgia* http://dx.doi.org/10.1177/0333102416630593 (2016).

[57] Sarchielli P, Corbelli I, Messina P et al (2016) Psychopathological comorbidities in medication-overuse headache: a multicentre clinical study. *Eur J Neurol* 23:85–91.https://doi.org/10.1111/ene.12794.

[58] Baumgartner C, Wessely P, Bingöl C et al (1989) Longterm prognosis of analgesic withdrawal in patients with drug-induced headaches. *Headache* 29: 510–514. https://doi.org/10.1111/j.1526-4610.1989.hed2908510.x

[59] Mathew NT, Stubits E, Nigam MP (1982) Transformation of episodic migraine into daily headache: analysis of factors. *Headache J Head Face Pain* 22: 66–68. https://doi.org/10.1111/j.1526-4610.1982.hed2202066.x

[60] Hagen K, Linde M, Steiner TJ et al (2012) Risk factors for medication-overuse headache: an 11-year follow-up study. The Nord-Trøndelag health studies. *Pain* 153:5661.https://doi.org/10.1016/j.pain.2011.08.018.

[61] Kristoffersen ES, Straand J, Russell MB, Lundqvist C (2016) Disability, anxiety and depression in patients with medication-overuse headache in primary care - the BIMOH study. *Eur J Neurol* 23:28–35.https://doi.org/10.1111/ene.12850.

[62] Bendtsen L, Munksgaard SB, Tassorelli C et al (2014) Disability, anxiety and depression associated with medication-overuse headache can be considerably reduced by detoxification and prophylactic treatment. Results from a multicentre, multinational study (COMOESTAS project). Cephalalgia 34: 426–433.https://doi.org/10.1177/0333102413515338.

[63] Lampl C, Thomas H, Tassorelli C et al (2016) Headache, depression and anxiety: associations in the Eurolight project. *J Headache Pain* 17(1):59.https://doi.org/10.1186/s10194-016-0649-2.

[64] Currone M, Tullo V, Mea E et al (2011) Psychopathological profile of patients with chronic migraine and medication overuse: study and findings in 50 cases. *Neurol Sci* 32:177-179. https://doi.org/10.1007/s10072-011-0527-2

[65] Cupini LM, Murtas MD, Costa C et al (2009) Obsessive-compulsive disorder and migraine with medication-overuse headache: research submission. *Headache* 49:1005-1013. https://doi.org/10.1111/j.1526-4610.2009.01457.x

[66] Radat F, Lanteri-Minet M (2010) What is the role of dependence-related behaviour in medication-overuse headache? Headache 50:1597–1611. https://doi.org/10.1111/j.1526-4610.2010.01755.x

[67] Galli F, Pozzi G, Frustaci A et al (2011) Differences in the personality

profile of medication-overuse headache sufferers and drug addict patients: a comparative study using MMPI-2. Headache 51:1212–1227.https://doi.org/10.1111/j.1526-4610.2011.01978.x

[68] He Z, Dong L, Zhang Y et al (2015) Metabolic syndrome in female migraine patients is associated with medication overuse headache: a clinic-based study in China. *Eur J Neurol* 22:1228–1234. https://doi.org/10.1111/ene.12732

[69] Westergaard ML, Glümer C, Hansen EH, Jensen RH (2016) Medication overuse, healthy lifestyle behaviour and stress in chronic headache: results from a population-based representative survey. *Cephalalgia* 36:15–28.https://doi.org/10.1177/0333102415578430.

[70] Sancisi E, Cevoli S, Vignatelli L et al (2010) Increased prevalence of sleep disorders in chronic headache: a case-control study. Headache 50:1464–1472. https://doi.org/10.1111/j.1526-4610.2010.01711.x

[71] Zeeberg P,Olesen J,Jensen R. Discontinuation of medication overuse in headache patients: recovery of therapeutic responsiveness.*Cephalalgia*2006;26:1192–1198. https://doi.org/10.1111/j.1468-2982.2006.01190.x

[72] Deiner et al *Cephalalgia* 2009(29) 1021-27 topiramate study.

[73] Does analgesic overuse matter? Response to OnabotulinumtoxinA in patients with chronic migraine with or without medication overuse Fayyaz Ahmed,Hassan W. Zafar,Alina Buture & Modar Khalil *SpringerPlus* **4**, Article number:589 (2015).

[74] Obermann M, Katsarava Z (2007) Management of medication overuse headache. Expert Rev Neurother 7:1145–1155, 10.1586/14737175.7.9.1145, 1:CAS: 528:DC%2BD2sXhtF2hsr7M, 17868013 DOI:10.1586/14737175.7.9.1145.

[75] Pamelaire K, Crevits L, Goadsby PJ, Haube H (2006) Practical management of medication overuse headache. Acta Neurol Belg 106:43–51

[76] Hering R, Steiner TJ (1991) Abrupt outpatient withdrawal of medication in analgesic abusers migraineurs. *Lancet* 337:1142–1443.

[77] Katsarava Z, Fritsche G, Muessig M, Diener HC, Limmroth V. Clinical features of withdrawal headache following overuse of triptans and other headache drugs. *Neurology*2001;57:1694–1698. https://doi.org.10.1212/wnl.57.9.1694

[78] Advice alone versus structured detoxification programmes for complicated medication overuse headache (MOH): a prospective, randomized, open-label trial Paolo Rossi, 1,2 Jessica Veronica Faroni,1Cristina Tassorelli,2and Giuseppe Nappi 2, *J Headache Pain*. 2013; 14(1): 10. Published online 2013 Feb 8. doi:10.1186/1129-2377-14-10.

[79] A Consensus Protocol for the Management of Medication-Overuse Headache: Evaluation in a Multicentric, Multinational Study, C Tassorelli R Jensen2,M Allena3,R De Icco4,G Sances3,Z Katsarava5,M Lainez6,Ja Leston7,R Fadic8,S Spadafora9,M Pagani10,G Nappi3 the COMOESTAS Consortium.2014 Aug;34(9):645-655. Cephalgia doi: 10.1177/0333102414521508.

[80] Complete Detoxification Is the Most Effective Treatment of Medication-Overuse Headache: A Randomized Controlled Open-Label Trial Louise Ninett Carlsen,Signe Bruun Munksgaard1,Rigmor Højland Jensen Lars Bendtsen12018 Feb;38(2):225-236. Doi: 10.1177/0333102417737779.

[81] Créac'h C, Frappe P, Cancade M et al (2011) In-patient versus out-patient withdrawal programmes for

medication overuse headache: a 2-year randomized trial. *Cephalalgia* 31: 1189-1198.https://doi.org/10.1177/0333102411412088.

[82] Zebenholzer K, Thamer M, Wöber C (2012) Quality of life, depression, and anxiety 6 months after inpatient withdrawal in patients with medication overuse headache: an observational study. *Clin J Pain* 28:284–290. https://doi.org/10.1097/AJP.0b013e3182321d35

[83] Grazzi L, Andrasik F, Usai S, Bussone G.In-patient vs. day-hospital withdrawal treatment for chronic migraine with medication overuse and disability assessment: results at one-year follow-up. *Neurol Sci* 2008; 29(Suppl.1): 161-163.

[84] Weatherall MW, Telzerow AJ, Cittadini E et al (2010) Intravenous aspirin (lysine acetylsalicylate) in the inpatient management of headache. *Neurology* 75(12):1098–1103.https://doi.org/10.1212/WNL.0b013e3181f39a11.

[85] Raskin NH (1986) Repetitive intravenous dihydroergotamine as therapy for intractable migraine. *Neurology* 36:995–997.https://doi.org/10.1212/WNL.36.7.995

[86] Mathew NT (1987) Amelioration of ergotamine withdrawal symptoms with naproxen. *Headache J Head Face Pain* 27: 130–133.https://doi.org/10.1111/j.1526-4610.1987.hed2703130.x

[87] Probyn K, Bowers H, Caldwell F et al (2017) Prognostic factors for chronic headache. *Neurology* 89:291–301. https://doi.org/10.1212/WNL.0000000000004112.

[88] Nagy AJ, Gandhi S, Bhola R, Goadsby PJ (2011) Intravenous dihydroergotamine for inpatient management of refractory primary headaches. *Neurology* 77(20):1827–1832. https:// doi.org/10.1212/WNL.0b013e3182377dbb.

[89] Cevoli Giannini G, Favoni V et al (2017) Treatment of withdrawal headache in patients with medication overuse headache: a pilot study. *J Headache* Pain.18(1):56.https://doi.org/10.1186/s10194-017-0763-9

[90] de Goffau MJ, Klaver ARE, Willemsen MG et al (2016) The effectiveness of treatments for patients with medication overuse headache; a systematic review and meta-analysis. *J Pain* 18:615–627.https://doi.org/10.1016/j.jpain.2016.12.005.

[91] Preventing and treating medication overuse headache Karl B. Alstadhaug, MD, PhD,a,b,*Hilde K. Ofte , MD, PhD, a and Espen S. Kristoffersen, MD, PhDc, dPain Rep. 2017 Jul; 2(4): Published online 2017 Jul 26. doi:10.1097/PR9.0000000000000612.

[92] Zeeberg P, Olesen J, Jensen R. Probable medication-overuse headache: the effect of a 2-month drug-free period. *Neurology* 2006; 6: 1894–1898.

[93] Deiner et al 2009 Cephalalgia, Hagen et al 2008 Cephalalgia, Ahmed et al Springerplus 2015, Silberstein et al 2013 The Journal of Neurological Sciences, Tepper et al Posters IHC Vancouver Erenumab works in both with or without medication overuse.

[94] Diener HC, Bussone G, Van Oene JC,Lahaye M,Schwalen S, Goadsby PJ; TOPMAT-MIG-201(TOP-CHROME) Study Group. Topiramate reduces headache days in chronic migraine: a randomized, double-blind, placebo-controlled study.*Cephalalgia* 2007; 27:814–823.

[95] Silberstein SD, Lipton RB, Dodick DW, *etal.*;Topiramate Chronic Migraine Study Group Efficacy and safety of topiramate for the treatment of chronic migraine: a randomized, double-blind, placebo-controlled trial. *Headache* 2007;47:170–180.

[96] Chiang C-C, Schwedt TJ, Wang S-J, Dodick DW (2016) Treatment of medication-overuse headache: a systematic review. *Cephalalgia* 36:371–386. https://doi.org/10.1177/0333102415593088

[97] Dodick DW, Turkel CC, DeGryse RE, *et al.* Onabotulinumtoxin A for treatment of chronic migraine: pooled results from the double-blind, randomized, placebo-controlled phases of the PREEMPT clinical program. *Headache* 2010; 50: 921–936.

[98] Prednisone as Initial Treatment of Analgesic-Induced Daily Headache A V Krymchantowski 1, J S Barbosa 2000 Mar;20(2):107-13 doi: 10.1046/j.1468-2982.2000.00028.x

[99] Prednisone vs. Placebo in Withdrawal Therapy Following Medication Overuse Headache L Pageler1,Z Katsarava,H C Diener,V Limmroth *Cephalgia* 2008 Feb; 28(2):152-6. doi: 10.1111/j.1468-2982.2007.01488.x.2007.

[100] Prednisolone Does Not Reduce Withdrawal Headache: A Randomized, Double-Blind StudyMagne G Bøe Ase Mygland,Rolf Salvesen 2007 Jul 3;69(1): 26 31.doi:10.1212/01.wnl.0000263652.46222.e8.

[101] Mitsikostas DD, Jumah MA. Medication overuse and headache. In: Martelletti P, editor. Handbook of headache. *Springer*, Milan; 2011. p. 638-50.

[102] Boes CJ, Black DF, Dodick DW. Pathophysiology and management of transformed migraine and medication overuse headache. Semin *Neurol* 2006; 26:232-41.

[103] Mathew NT. Amelioration of ergotamine withdrawal symptoms with naproxen. *Headache* 1987;27:130-3.

[104] Probyn K, Bowers H, Caldwell F et al (2017) Prognostic factors for chronic headache: a systematic review. *Neurology* 89:291–301.

[105] Diener HC, Dichgans J, Scholz E et al (1989) Analgesic-induced chronic headache: long-term results of withdrawal therapy. *J Neurol* 236:9–14. https://doi.org/10.1007/BF00314210

[106] Suhr B, Evers S, Bauer B et al (1999) Drug-induced headache: long-term results of stationary versus ambulatory withdrawal therapy. *Cephalalgia* 19:44–49.

[107] Schnider P, Aull S, Baumgartner C et al (1996) Long-term outcome of patients with headache and drug abuse after inpatient withdrawal: five-year follow-up. *Cephalalgia* 16:481–485.

[108] Fritsche G, Eberl A, Katsarava Z et al (2001) Drug-induced headache: long-term follow-up of withdrawal therapy and persistence of drug misuse. *Eur Neurol* 45:229–235.https://doi.org/10.1159/000052134.

[109] Grazzi L, Andrasik F, D'Amico D et al (2002) Behavioral and pharmacologic treatment of transformed migraine with analgesic overuse: outcome at 3 years. *Headache* 42:483–490.https://doi.org/10.1046/j.1526-4610.2002.02123.x

[110] Zidverc-Trajkovic J, Pekmezovic T, Jovanovic Z et al (2007) Medication overuse headache: clinical features predicting treatment outcome at 1-year follow-up. *Cephalalgia* 27:1219–1225. https://doi.org/10.1111/j.1468-2982.2007.01432.x

[111] Bigal ME, Rapoport AM, Sheftell FD et al (2004) Transformed migraine and medication overuse in a tertiary headache Centre–clinical characteristics and treatment outcomes. *Cephalalgia an Int J headache* 24:483–490. https://doi.org/10.1111/j.1468-2982.2004.00691.x

[112] Sances G, Galli F, Anastasi S et al (2010) Medication-overuse headache

and personality: a controlled study by means of the MMPI-2: research submission. *Headache* 50:198–209. https://doi.org/10.1111/ j.1526-4610.2009.01593.x

[113] Bøe MG, Salvesen R, Mygland Å (2009) Chronic daily headache with medication overuse: predictors of outcome 1 year after withdrawal therapy. *Eur J Neurol* 16:705–712. https://doi.org/10.1111/ j.1468-1331.2009.02571.x

[114] Bøe MG, Thortveit E, Vatne A, Mygland Å (2017) Chronic headache with medication overuse: long-term prognosis after withdrawal therapy. *Cephalalgia* 37:1215–1221. https://doi. org/10.1177/0333102416672493

[115] Zidverc-Trajkovic JJ, Pekmezovic T, Jovanovic Z et al (2016) Long-term predictors of remission in patients treated for medication-overuse headache at a specialized headache center: a prospective cohort study. *Cephalalgia* 0:1–9.https://doi.org/ 10.1177/0333102416683918.

[116] Zeeberg P, Olesen J, Jensen R (2006) Discontinuation of medication overuse in headache patients: recovery of therapeutic responsiveness. *Cephalalgia* 26:1192–1198.https://doi. org/10.1111/j.1468-2982.2006.01190.x

[117] Evers S, Suhr B, Bauer B et al (1999) A retrospective long-term analysis of the epidemiology and features of drug-induced headache. *J Neurol* 246:802–809.https://doi.org/ 10.1007/s004150050458.

[118] Katsarava Z, Limmroth V, Finke M et al (2003) Rates and predictors for relapse in medication overuse headache: a 1-year prospective study. *Neurology* 60: 1682–1683.

[119] Sances G, Ghiotto N, Galli F et al (2010) Risk factors in medication-overuse headache: a 1-year follow-up study (care II protocol). Cephalalgia 30: 329–336. https://doi.org/10.1111/ j.1468-2982.2009.01934.x

[120] Jensen RH, Bendtsen L (2008) Medication overuse headache in Scandinavia. *Cephalalgia* 28:1237–1239.

[121] Medication Overuse Headache: Rates and Predictors for Relapse in a 4-year Prospective Study Z Katsarava1, M Muessig, A Dzagnidze, G Fritsche, H C Diener, V Limmroth *Cephalgia* 2005 Jan;25(1):12-5.

[122] Comparison of 3 Treatment Strategies for Medication Overuse Headache. *JAMA Neurology* doi:10.1001/ jamaneurol.2020.1179 https:// jamanetwork.com/full article/2766518.